The International Library of Psychology

THE LAWS OF FEELING

T0264799

Founded by C. K. Ogden

The International Library of Psychology

PHYSIOLOGICAL PSYCHOLOGY
In 10 Volumes

THE LAWS OF FEELING

F PAULHAN

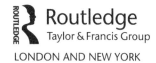

LONDON AND NEW YORK

First published in 1930
by Routledge, Trench, Trubner & Co., Ltd.
2 Park Square, Milton Park, Abingdon, Oxfordshire OX14 4RN
711 Third Avenue, New York, NY 10017

First issued in paperback 2014

Routledge is an imprint of the Taylor and Francis Group, an informa business

© 1930 F Paulhan, Translated by C K Ogden

British Library Cataloguing in Publication Data
A CIP catalogue record for this book
is available from the British Library

The Laws of Feeling
ISBN 0415-21079-8
Physiological Psychology: 10 Volumes
ISBN 0415-21131-X
The International Library of Psychology: 204 Volumes
ISBN 0415-19132-7

ISBN 13: 978-1-138-88258-4 (pbk)
ISBN 13: 978-0-415-21079-9 (hbk)

CONTENTS

v

CONTENTS

PREFACE

THOUGH it cannot be said that the writings of Frédéric Paulhan are entirely unknown outside France, references to his name in English publications are few and far between.[1] Already, however, before the War he had been responsible for more than a dozen major works, and in 1928-9 his latest treatises, *Les Puissances de l'Abstraction* and *La Double Fonction du Langage*, completed a twenty-volume programme whose main features were determined over sixty years ago.

Paulhan, in fact, has been one of the leading figures in contemporary psychology for over half-a-century. So early as 1877 he began to contribute important articles to the *Revue Philosophique*. In 1880 appeared his *Physiologie de l'Esprit*, in which year Ribot referred to his original treatment of emotion, and expressed his general agreement with Paulhan's views.[2] And in the latest achievement of the French school, the monumental *Traité de Psychologie* (1923-4), Paulhan's conclusions on the subject of feeling are accepted as fundamental,[3] while the debt of modern French psychology to his work as a whole is emphasized by Professor Dumas in his final summary.[4]

[1] *L'Activité mentale* is referred to by Stout (*Analytic Psychology*, Vol. II, pp. 116, 133), by Ward (*Psychological Principles*, p. 309), who points out certain relationships to Herbart, and by Shand (*Foundations of Character*, p. 21), who also makes use of Paulhan's work on Character ; Baldwin (*Thought and Things*, Vol. III) is indebted to the *Mensonge* series ; but all are concerned with isolated minor features.

[2] *Revue Philosophique*, 1880, p. 570.

[3] Vol. I, p. 464.

[4] Vol. II, p. 1140—" C'est de plus une justice à rendre à la psychoogie synthétiste, et particulièrement a celle de Paulhan, qu'elle a abouti à nous représenter l'esprit comme une réalité vivante. . . ." In a word, the solid achievement of Taine was adapted by Paulhan to the needs of another century.

The original of the present volume was first published in 1884 in the *Revue Philosophique* under the title *Les phénomènes affectifs, et les lois de leur apparition*. It was enlarged in book form in 1887. A second edition was called for in 1901, and a third in 1912, but for many years before the fourth edition appeared (1926) it remained, like so much of the best French psychology, out of print and unobtainable. There is no copy in the Bodleian, the London University Library, the London Library, the Science Museum Library, or the Psychological Library at Cambridge. The edition of 1901 may, however, be found in the British Museum and that of 1887 in the Cambridge University Library. This work has here been supplemented, with his consent, by M. Paulhan's contribution to the *Revue Philosophique* (July-August, 1920, Nos. 7-8) entitled "La sensibilité, l'intelligence et la volonté dans tous les faits psychologiques".

The translation itself was begun at a time when the challenge of Endocrinology, Behaviorism, and the various branches of Comparative Physiology, no less than the successful advance of Psycho-analysis, made it seem doubtful to many whether psychology ought not shortly to dispense with psychologists, in the traditional sense, altogether. It was therefore laid circumspectly aside until, after a lapse of ten years, it became clear that the more advanced members of a variety of schools were converging on a formulation closely resembling that to which so much thought had already been given by others of whose very existence they were presumably unaware.[1]

Moreover, if it be true, as Professor Lashley told the Ninth International Congress of Psychology (1929), that "psychology is to-day a more fundamental science

---

[1] It is worth recalling that in 1894-5 John Dewey elaborated in the *Psychological Review* a theory of emotion as an overflow of energy into the viscera—in the physiological terminology of the Lange-James theory. Cf. also Janet, *L'état mentale des Hystériques* (1911), pp. 543-4.

than neurophysiology ", there are branches of psychology
in which the decade 1930-40 has something to learn
from the still more fundamental science prevalent under
the same name in 1880-90.   " By this I mean," continues
the President of the American Psychological Association, "that the latter offers few principles from which
we may predict or define the normal organization
of behaviour, whereas the study of psychological processes furnishes a mass of factual material to which the
laws of nervous reaction in behaviour must conform."[1]
For the modern psychologist, however, "the problem of
emotion is still in such confusion that one can draw no
conclusions with confidence."

Paulhan's main thesis, that feeling and emotion are
due to an arrest of tendencies, may be related historically
to the suggestions of Bain and Maudsley to which
reference is made on pages 24 and 44.   The treatment
of emotion as due to the overflow consequent on this
arrest may to-day commend itself to many who would
hesitate to extend it to the whole affective field.
Paulhan's generalization of the law to cover all forms
of feeling, including both pleasure and pain as he
defines them (pp. 19 and 82), is implicit in the very
broad bio-physical conception of man as an un-
adapted animal (p. 191) which also underlies his theory
of consciousness (p. 10) and personality (p. 144).

That such an approach to psychological phenomena,
whatever its ultimate validity, may be fruitful in the
development of new lines of thought is shown by
reference to other works in the Library of Psychology.
Thus the reader of Vaihinger's *Philosophy of As-if* will
find (*infra* pp. 176-9) a full awareness of the heuristic
value of error, while Professor Thurstone's account of
The Nature of Intelligence and Rignano's explanation of
rational and representative processes in his *Psychology of
Reasoning* are foreshadowed in the discussions of the

---

[1] K. S. Lashley, *The Psychological Review*, January 1930 : a passage
which the curious may compare with pages 11-12 of the present work.

selective character of intelligence (p. 111) and its adaptive, experimental function (p. 176) respectively. The main contention of those who adopt the *Gestalt* terminology will be recognized in the account of the relation of a feeling to its constituent parts (pp. 132-4), while material for a sane development of Behaviorism might have been derived from the remarks on observation and introspection at page 11. Moreover, since the first great disturbance of equilibrium, and the first arrest of the fundamental tendency of the organism thereto, is due to *The Trauma of Birth*, even the speculations of Dr Rank might have found an impressive setting in a theory which accounts so plausibly both for Anxiety and for Excitement. Psycho-analysis in general may also profit by the neutral treatment of Adaptation and Adjustment; on page 95, for example, will be found an account of organic disturbance due to emotional conflict, successfully freed (cf. p. 144) from the moral and political interpretations to which the neo-Adlerian movement is so naïvely prone.

It is significant, too, that an able modern writer on thalamo-cortical relations goes so far as to attribute Paulhan's basic doctrine to a recent volume on *The Psychology of Emotion* in the Library itself:—

"Dr McCurdy links emotion intimately and indissolubly with instinct, from which emotion is developed. This development takes place in three stages. First, if the organism responds to a stimulus immediately and adequately with instinctive behaviour, no emotion whatever is engendered. Secondly, if the instinctive reaction be held up, emotional expression and, if the subject be self-conscious, some affect will appear. The latter represents what is not expressed in any way. Thirdly occurs a stage in which affect alone appears, which is as poignant as the emotion is purely subjective." [1]

From the point of view of observation, continues Mr Diblee, "this analysis must be regarded as having very great authority, particularly in respect of regarding

---

[1] G. B. Diblee, *Instinct and Intuition*, 1929, p. 213.

emotion as to some extent a storm of expression, or self-expression, which is alternative to instinctive activity."
What is perhaps even more surprising is that the same author, interpreting this view to mean that "instinct is the sole source of emotion",[1] objects at some length that emotions may have intellectual elements. The upshot resembles a controversy in which pages 150-156 of the present work should appear as the contribution of a critic of the first 84 pages.

Upholders of the Double-language[2] solution of the Mind-Body problem will find much to agree with in Paulhan's discussion of psychical and physical on pages 10 and 56, as well as in the criticisms of the Double-aspect theory on page 8. But it is in the domain of Æsthetics[3] that the general treatment of feeling and tendency here developed is likely to prove most significant. It provides a valuable theoretical background for the doctrine of Equilibrium and Synæsthesis in support of which various passages in Schiller, Coleridge, and Sully have been cited, though it can hardly be said to have received explicit recognition till recent years.

But, it may be felt, supposing all this to be true,

[1] On page 217 he even suggests that instinct and emotion are identified, though on page 17 McCurdy's explicit statement (p. 87) that they are alternative phenomena ("emotional expressions must be viewed as secondary manifestations of instincts which appear when the primary behaviour is inhibited from any cause"—*i.e.* if tendencies are not arrested there is no emotion) is characterized as admitting that the relations between them "are more apparent than real". The statement, however, that if food is properly digested no dyspepsia occurs neither implies that the relation between meals and stomach-aches, or assimilation and nausea, is more apparent than real, nor yet does it make that relation one of identity.

[2] The view that we are concerned essentially with two symbol systems rather than with parallel processes, with aspects, or with situations requiring labels such as 'idealism' or 'materialism'. Cf. Pièron, *Thought and the Brain* (Introduction), and the linguistic approach of the present writer and Professor I. A. Richards in *The Meaning of Meaning* (3rd Edition, 1930, p. 22).

[3] See especially page 24; and cf. *Encyclopædia Britannica* (1926 Supplementary Volumes—13th Edition), *sub.* " Æsthetics ".

supposing his fundamental thesis to be acceptable, would not a Paulhan fifty years younger be concerning himself to-day with other material, other problems?

The answer seems to be that, in the precise and rather special field which has here been selected, there would probably be no need for any very significant re-orientation. There might be more attention to the technical literature of *repression* and the *complex*, of *motor consciousness* and the *typological* method, of the *thalamus* and the *endocrines;* and according to temperament or equipment a modern author might find himself referring to Cannon[1] and Crookshank,[2] to Köhler[3] and Kretschmer,[4] to Marston[5] and Miller,[6] to Pavlov[7] and Pièron[8] rather than to Taine and Bain. In addition, from *Feelings and Emotions (The Wittenberg Symposium)*, 1928, it could be demonstrated that a quorum of the world's most eminent psychologists, wrangling for six days on the Laws of Feeling, often found themselves in substantial agreement with Paulhan (cf. pp. 63, 126-8, 235, 309, etc.) — though his name was never mentioned. If, therefore, the student is prepared to follow up these clues, he is not likely to be led astray by any failure of the *Zeitgeist* to accommodate itself to the 'eighties in every respect.

Paulhan, moreover, is one of a small group of writers whose linguistic conscience is so acute that they avoid the major errors of verbalism which subsequent controversy may either remove or enlarge into doctrine. Descriptively therefore he still tells us just what he wished to say ; and all sensitive analytic description retains its value.

[1] For physiological phenomena—*Bodily Changes in Pain, Hunger, Fear and Rage* (1915).

[2] For emotional neuroses—*Migraine* (1926).

[3] For animal emotivity—*The Mentality of Apes* (1925).

[4] For physical types—*Physique and Character* (1925).

[5] For motor consciousness—*The Emotions of Normal People* (1928).

[6] For neurological parallels—*The Integrative Action of the Mind* (1931).

[7] For inhibition and conditioning—*The Conditioned Reflex* (1929).

[8] For all the latest news—*Principles of Experimental Psychology* 1929).

One of the most valuable results of a consistent theory of feeling would be the possibility of progress on the symbolic side, both as regards a scientific notation and for purposes of linguistic simplification. Whether we are dealing with the 54 feelings mentioned by Titchener, the 70 distinguished by Messer, or the 1300 envisaged by Dr Gruehn of Berlin—of which he has already listed 575!—some sort of ordering principle is necessary if our analyses are to have more value than an account of the shapes of clouds or flints. Until recently some method such as that of Shand has seemed to many psychologists the most hopeful. For others the equally fundamental work of Marston now also holds out a dim prospect of advance. A third approach is suggested by the parallel need for a notation of colour, and it is significant that the emotional aspect of colour is one on which Marston has laid stress, while Paulhan not only accepts the analogy (pp. 108, 121) but his general theory (especially pp. 65 and 82) suggests the possibility of quantitative gradations ordering the whole affective range. It is a long way from the cat on the hearth enjoying a 'feeling of warmth', via the 'man of feeling' and the 'feeling of envy', to the musician 'overcome by intense feeling' or the 'deep feelings of awe and reverence' with which literature abounds. Psychologists profess themselves embarrassed by the ambiguity ; yet if it were a valid generalization, it is no more surprising than that which allows both science and commonsense to cover everything from a Pekinese to a St Bernard by the unlikely caption 'dog'. But whereas the zoologist has proceeded to regularize his canine notation, the psychologist is still searching for the differentia of his affective species. Paulhan's claims to have provided a systematizing criterion are therefore particularly worthy of consideration.

The phraseology of French affective psychology undoubtedly has its demerits from the standpoint of the translator ; but it is hoped that sufficient of the spirit of the original has been preserved to enable the clarity of the author's thought as well as the subtle and sinuous spiral of his exegetic to make their due appeal. In general the terminology has been closely followed, the only important deviation being that which appears in the title itself. The term Feeling is, however, here used in what may be regarded as its orthodox sense both in psychology and in common parlance.[1]

C. K. O.

[1] Cf. Stout, *Analytic Psychology*, Vol. I, p. 121—" We therefore agree with Professor James in giving a very wide application to the word ' feeling '. We must however steadfastly refuse to make it cover sensation and thought indifferently, as he appears to do "—and as Professor Thorndike certainly does (*Elements of Psychology*, 1917, pp. 4-7). " There is," continues Stout, " no generic term in ordinary language which comprehends both pleasure and pain, and nothing besides ; " a restriction of the term ' feeling ' to what others call ' feeling-tone ' (algedonics) is, however, characteristic of the third main terminological group.

THE LAWS OF FEELING

INTRODUCTORY

I

I PROPOSE in this work to discuss the general psychology of feeling. The undertaking will doubtless seem ambitious, and perhaps premature. The problem is one of those that psychologists have studied least.

If we compare what we know about the intellect with what we know about feeling, it is evident that the advances of psychology are immeasurably greater in all that appertains to the purely intellectual side of the human mind. Our information concerning the general laws of knowledge, and some of their particular forms such as memory, imagination, perception and reasoning, is considerable ; many facts have been observed, grouped and co-ordinated, and a number of theories may be considered as definitive. The laws of feeling, on the other hand, are very little known ; certain particular forms of sensibility, the moral sense, the religious sense, and the æsthetic sense, have been studied with some care, especially in their outward manifestations and their social effects ; we also have many theories relating to pleasure and pain, and there are interesting books on the emotions and passions ; but the results cannot be compared with those obtained in other psychological fields ; while upon the nature, causes, and activity of the feelings in general little light has been thrown, apart from the laws which also apply to all other psychical phenomena.

The laws which I shall endeavour to determine in this volume are those connected with the appearance

A   1

of affective phenomena. I shall first discuss the conditions and general characters of these phenomena ;
then the particular modifications of those general conditions which give rise to each of the principal groups
of feelings ; and, finally, the laws of the manifestation
of compound feelings, that is to say, the relations of
affects to the affective or non-affective elements which
give rise to them. But as we must refer these laws
to general psychology, and determine the place of feeling in the general working of the mind, it is worth
while to establish or recall the psychological principles
that should serve as a basis for the inquiry, before we
proceed to discuss these various questions.

II

Man is an ensemble of organs united and harmonized by one of those organs, the nervous system ;
the unity which he possesses is maintained by the
systematization of his organs—an imperfect but real
systematization. Man may therefore be considered
as an ensemble, an incompletely organized complex of
organico - psychical systems : the main systems are
broken up into secondary systems, and these again
into others of less importance. All these systems may
interpenetrate and combine with one another or be
broken up. The same element may appear in many
different systems, and the same system may combine
with other systems to form varied complexes of a higher
order, or may break up and dissociate into a number
of parts, which severally combine with different systems.
Thus, for example, the system of images of various
kinds, of signs and movements, which constitutes the
letter *a*, may unite with various other systems of images
and movements to produce in us the images of different
words. Each word can be associated with other words
to form a more complex system, a phrase ; while, from
a different point of view, a word set in a phrase is

decomposed and loses some of its elements. A word which is understood by the mind is associated with numerous ideas and obscure interpretations ; and, according to the meaning of its context, not all of those constructions and ideas, but only a few among them, are evoked. Thus, the word *letter* will not call forth the same psychological state, will not be associated with the same ideas, when it occurs in a phrase relating to correspondence, as when it occurs in a sentence about the alphabet.[1] These few examples, which could be multiplied *ad infinitum*, are sufficient to show the general mechanism of psychical systems. Human life is only a continual association and dissociation of elements and systems : the more the elements combine into systems, and the more these systems are co-ordinated, the more closely man approaches perfection, but this co-ordination can often only be effected by means of previous dissociations. To essay a general psychology of feeling, then, is to seek out what particular relations of psychical elements or systems generate the affective phenomena, and what part these phenomena play, when once they are produced, either by their own influence, or, more probably, by that of the physiological processes which accompany them, in the organization of the individual. I shall only attempt to deal with the first part of this task in the present volume.

But man is not only a system, or rather an ensemble of systems : he is a systematizing system. He extends the harmony which exists in himself over the world to which he owes it—perhaps wholly, at any rate partially —by adapting to some single purpose natural objects which, without him, would remain isolated from one another and lacking all harmonious connection. This is what he is doing when, for example, he takes iron and coal from the earth, wood from trees, skins from animals, glass, and the materials made from various

[1] See Bréal's study, "Comment les mots s'associent dans notre esprit", published in the *Revue politique et littéraire*.

natural objects, and works upon them and other things, modifies them, and finally combines them to produce a system of rails, locomotives and carriages. Man is a sort of ferment of systematization, and, consequently, of morality, introduced into the world. This systematization, moreover, comes about through the medium of the nervous system. It establishes, as Spencer showed, the adaptation of man to his environment; and we must add that, perhaps to the same extent, it serves to adapt the environment to man. By these successive adaptations, when circumstances are favourable, there is formed a system which, at any rate in some respects, becomes less and less imperfect, in that it comprises more parts and the parts are more closely linked together in view of one supreme end or of particular harmonious ends.

In this vast complex, which includes, as may be seen, inorganic elements, organized and animate beings, and men, there are many centres. Of these man is the chief—we may here consider man in general as an individual, and need not concern ourselves with social complexes—and in man we are dealing with the nervous system. He receives impressions from without, dissociates them, analyses them, and classifies them as a whole; classifies their elements, unites them anew, either collectively or in their elements, with a host of other elements, similar or different, to form the psychical systems of which we have spoken; and he reacts according to his own nature. Some of his reactions are general, others are particular: the former are derived from general properties of the nervous tissue, or, if we prefer to put it so, they are phenomena which appear wherever those other phenomena that make up what is called the nervous system are present; the latter vary with individuals and groups of individuals. The first are the reactions of a genus or species; the second are individual. There are, moreover, all possible gradations between the one and the other. Certain reactions are common to all healthy men ; for instance, the reflex action which makes the pupil dilate or contract, according to the degree of intensity of a light-stimulus ; others are met with only in a given section of mankind ; among cannibals impressions upon the senses due to human bodies are, in certain circumstances, followed by appropriate reactions leading to the cooking and eating of the said bodies. This reaction is no longer produced, or reappears only very rarely, and in extreme circumstances, among civilized peoples. Thus there are reactions which are proper to certain races of men, or to certain ages ; while others result from conditions of sex or occupation, or from a particular idiosyncrasy, and are purely individual. The more or less harmonious grouping of these reactions, due to genus, species, tribe, age, sex, heredity, to special physical structure and to the general or particular circumstances in which the organism exists or happens to be placed, makes up what we style the character or the individuality of each of us.

These diverse reactions of the nervous system to the various excitations received from the external or internal world belong to the type of reflex action, taking the word in its widest sense. This is the only theory compatible with the universal determinism of phenomena, which, if it be not absolutely demonstrated, certainly appears to be supported by the most probable inductions of the various sciences and of psychology in particular. If there have been some partial and apparent exceptions, if we admit a spontaneity such as that discussed by Bain, which is not contrary to determinism, this is clearly unimportant ; for, on the one hand, the nervous system is always, in a sense, subject to external conditions, and, moreover, such a spontaneity can be referred to a formula similar to that which expresses the general characters of other phenomena of human activity, provided that this formula is made a little more comprehensive than has been usual.

So far, we have spoken only of the nervous system, and not of intelligence or feeling ; we must now explain ourselves upon this point, and elucidate the nature of the part played by consciousness. One consideration which immediately presents itself enables us to assign to it, at the most, a secondary importance as regards human systematization. Consciousness, in fact, is frequently absent from the nerve reactions which occur in organized beings. In man, for instance, the reflex action of the spinal cord produces no psychical phenomenon which can be observed by the individual consciousness. The reflex actions of the spine are not alone in this respect. We are therefore obliged to recognize that consciousness is not a condition necessary to the harmony of the organs. The vegetative life should be sufficient to prove this. Consequently we are not bound to explain purpose by intelligence ; the conjunction of several phenomena or of several processes conducing to one end or to harmonious ends is not in the least indicative of a conscious cause, as people are pleased to believe ; and upon a little reflection it is clear that there is absolutely nothing in consciousness itself which can entitle us to endow it with that property of organization and systematization which we refuse to matter.

An easily explainable but wholly irrational association usually leads people to see in intelligence a necessary antecedent to phenomena whose grouping discloses a sort of unity. There is no good reason why intelligence, as a psychical fact, should possess a co-ordinating power which nothing else could have. For how can the idea of a complex fact be one of the conditions of that fact, or why must a complex fact be preceded by the mental representation of that fact? No good reason can be given for this, unless it be that experience does show us that in certain circumstances the notion of an action precedes the action, and that the idea of an intricate object precedes the object itself. But experience by no means authorizes us to deduce a law from this, since there is nothing in the analysis of the law to indicate that the elements are logically connected among themselves, and since, on the other hand, examples of complicated and co-ordinated actions caused without the intervention of intelligence are very numerous, although for reasons easy to understand man may be less prone to observe and take account of them. Confining ourselves to indications furnished by man, it is clear that the nervous system produces purposive action without the intervention of consciousness, and that purpose is never realized by consciousness without the intervention of the nervous system. We must, therefore, in our general conception of man, from the very first attribute a preponderant influence to nervous activity in relation to consciousness.

" Physiology ", said Ribot, speaking of the conscious state, "teaches us that its production is always connected with the state of the nervous system, especially of the brain. But the converse is not true; if all psychical activity implies nervous activity, not all nervous activity implies psychical activity. Nervous activity is therefore much more widespread than psychical activity; consciousness is something superadded."

We come then to a conception of man as an imperfect system of organs linked together by the nervous system, and brought into harmony (a harmony equally imperfect) with other similar systems, as well as with the physical world, by this same nervous system ; and we notice that certain of the processes of adaptation which occur in a part of this nervous system are accompanied by a particular kind of phenomena called states of consciousness. Everything leads us to believe a priori that these play no essential part in the process of adaptation and systematization ; it is necessary to examine more closely whether this is indeed the case.

Ribot has clearly formulated and discussed the question

in the chapter from which I have just quoted.[1] He ranges himself, with some qualifications, on the side of the psychologists who regard consciousness as a phenomenon merely accompanying certain reflex cerebral acts. But Ribot concedes to consciousness more importance than the partisans of this theory generally allow. The view which I am about to state here is, I believe, somewhat different from Maudsley's theory of automatism, as well as from that of Ribot. At any rate, it approaches the question in a somewhat different way. It may be that we are dealing in fine shades of difference, but it is the more necessary to give precision to questions according as they are more complex and delicate ; and it has been said with reason that subtlety is essential to the psychologist.

According to all the data of psychology, we are justified in the belief that every phenomenon of consciousness is accompanied by a physiological phenomenon. The problem is to discover the relation that exists between the psychical and the physical. Men have tried to explain the psychical and the physical as two aspects or manifestations of a single substance. Explanations of this character have one grave defect— they do not explain anything ; as is always the case when the idea of substance is introduced. I do not wish here to go deeply into the question from a philosophical point of view, or in the light of general criticism ; it will be sufficient to say a few words in explanation of what is necessary to psychology, reserving the ultimate interpretation.

Experience and induction, then, give us two parallel series of phenomena ; one series is constant, the other exists only in certain conditions and is frequently interrupted.

Suppose by way of hypothesis that the second or incomplete series is suppressed, the other remaining as before ; the actions of the man will be absolutely the

[1] Ribot, *Les Maladies de la personnalité*, Introduction, 1885.

same, in point of fact, and will be determined by an unconscious physiological process instead of by a physiological process with attendant conscious phenomena. I am well aware that such an hypothesis is actually inadmissible, since, if the desired physiological conditions were present, consciousness must necessarily be produced, but it involves nothing that cannot be easily imagined. It must be allowed, of course, that for the actions to be precisely the same, the physiological conditions must be identical—including even the peculiarities, still partly unknown, which are the physiological conditions of consciousness. What in fact constitutes the rôle of consciousness, and its importance for the development of psychical life—an importance which Ribot has emphasized in the chapter already mentioned—is not the phenomenon of consciousness itself, but more properly the series of particular physiological conditions which accompany it and which are the appropriate conditions of consciousness, namely, the quantity and quality of the blood, the duration and complexity of the act, etc. If we imagine all the physiological conditions of the conscious act to be present, we can very well conceive that consciousness may be suppressed without loss for the external manifestation of personality. It would obviously be no longer the same if the particular conditions of consciousness were wanting, and if, instead of a physico-psychological fact, we had a merely physiological fact ; but if this change modified the result, and lessened its importance, that would not be because the second process was attended by consciousness whereas the first was without that accompaniment, but because the two processes would differ from one another physiologically. " It follows from the hypothesis ", says Ribot, " that since the conscious state involves more numerous, or at any rate other, physiological conditions than the unconscious, two individuals, one coming under the first head and the other under the second, are, other things being equal, not strictly comparable." In my opinion, it is this physiological difference which is important and is sufficient to give rise to all the other differences—though we may see these differences in their psychological aspect and so attribute them to consciousness itself, when there may really be no other cause than the physiological process. In opposition, therefore, to the partisans of an over-simple automatism, I admit that a purely physiological process and a psycho-physiological process are not equivalent from the mental point of view, but I maintain that the difference between the two processes is due, not to the fact that the one is accompanied by consciousness, but to the physiological differences which distinguish them,[1] consciousness being merely a sign of those differences.

We need not conclude from the above that consciousness is only of secondary importance in the study of psychology. It is easy to see that it must be otherwise. Indeed, we have admitted as a preliminary answer, without prejudice to the philosophical solution of the problem, that the phenomena of consciousness form a sort of parallel process, in certain conditions, to the physiological process. Now it is this physiological or psycho-physiological process, beginning with a sensation and ending with an action, which is the subject of psychology, or at any rate of its central part. But it

---

[1] I am fully aware of one of the philosophical objections that may be brought against this conception of consciousness. In the main, it is that consciousness is reduced to playing only a minor part in the world, that it becomes indifferent, with no useful function, and would tend, it may be, to disappear, and to give place to a complete automatism ; yet we can know nothing save conscious acts, and we have no possible mode of existence other than as states of consciousness. The brain and the nervous system are only known to us in facts of consciousness of a certain kind, and we ought perhaps not to attribute to them a reality 'in themselves', apart from any conscious form. I believe that there is a reply to these objections, but this is not the place to pursue the subject ; it is better to avoid complications, if possible. We can for the moment be content to take things as they present themselves in psychology, reserving, as was remarked above, the final interpretation which belongs to general philosophy.

is precisely this phase of the process which is most difficult of access for physiological observation, and frequently it can only be suspected or guessed at by inference ; it also happens to be that part which is frequently accompanied by consciousness. We at once see, therefore, the utility of these phenomena to us, for they are parallel to the processes which we are investigating, and can inform us as to their direction, their intensity, their associations, etc. In short, as there is no fact of consciousness which does not correspond to a physiological fact, and as the two are connected by precise laws, we cannot study one without at the same time studying the other. Every psychological study is a physiological study, and we study the brain by studying the facts of consciousness, exactly as we inform ourselves as to a man's intelligence by listening to his words, which are its observable signs. As in many other cases, one means of knowing may be substituted for another. If, for example, we live near a railway, we can tell by the noise if a train is passing and even whether it is a goods train, an ordinary train, or an express. Auditory sensations take the place of visual sensations, and the second can be inferred from the first. Similarly, when we experience any sensation we can argue from what is perceived by the inner sense to the visual or other phenomena which we commonly call nervous, and which could be observed if we had adequate means of investigation. The procedure is the same. In studying psycho-physiological phenomena through consciousness, we are like deaf-mutes who can guess by lip-reading the words they do not hear.

These considerations, in my opinion, allow us to be more daring in our interpretation than the facts of nerve physiology might authorize. Once we know the general modes of nervous activity and the general relations of this nervous activity to psychic activity, we can, I think, draw inferences, at any rate if we proceed on general lines, and from a given order of phenomena, the psychical, arrive at phenomena of another order, which are not directly known. I do not say that there is nothing hypothetical in this method of procedure, but it would be easy to prove by cogent arguments that everything which can be known is to some extent hypothetical, and in my opinion the process of which I speak does not exceed the limits of legitimate hypothesis.

CHAPTER I

THE GENERAL LAW OF THE PRODUCTION OF FEELING

I. *The arrest of tendencies*

EVERY emotion, every feeling, every pleasure or pain, has its particular conditions of existence, which always produce it and no other state. But if we consider these phenomena as constituting one and the same group of facts, we shall recognize that the same general law manifests itself in each particular case where one of them is produced ; they are all subject to common conditions, which correspond to what they possess in common in spite of their differences—to that something which differentiates them, for instance, from a purely intellectual phenomenon, or from any physical phenomenon. To inquire into the particular conditions which give rise to such and such an emotion, to such and such a feeling, is the business of special psychology ; to inquire into the general conditions which always give rise to some phenomenon of the affective order, and can only give rise to such a phenomenon, is our present task.

With a view to determining these conditions and setting forth the law which expresses them, we may avail ourselves of the double method of analysis and synthesis. We shall first take an obviously affective phenomenon, and by analysis of the various conditions of its production we shall ascertain, with the help of experience, which among those conditions are essential and correspond to its peculiar affective property. Their character will be clearly shown if their disappearance, the other conditions remaining unaltered, causes the disappearance of the affective character of the phenomenon in question, while its remaining characters undergo no change. Inversely, experience will show by what change of antecedents an affective phenomenon can take the place of some intellectual phenomenon which may closely resemble it except in so far as the particular affective quality is concerned.

Mere observation of conscious acts and their development is of itself enough to give good indications and to supply us with a great number of phenomena whence the law in question may be derived. We shall note at an early stage that physiological research and pathological records confirm the results which may be drawn from the direct observations made by ourselves or by others. Habit, which so greatly alters psychical phenomena, and as a general rule diminishes the emotional factor, enables us easily to see how this transformation is effected. To take a common example, which every one has had an opportunity of observing : the effects of shyness. Imagine a man, timid to excess, making a first call upon people whom he knows very slightly or not at all. Affective phenomena are in this case abundant—emotions of regret, embarrassment, boredom, a feeling of apprehension, and sometimes of curiosity, etc. If the action is repeated frequently, these affective phenomena generally vanish, except in particular circumstances which we may neglect in order not to complicate our account, and if there be no reason for the production of new or different feelings, they are replaced by a mechanical indifference.

We have here, therefore, two groups of almost identical phenomena, resembling one another at least externally ; but however close we suppose this resemblance to be, there appears in the first group an ensemble of affective phenomena which is absent from the second. The whole problem is to discover what changes in the causes have brought about this change in the effects, and which conditions have disappeared in the second case. We are here concerned, of course, only with psycho-physiological conditions and need not take into account outside circumstances which, moreover, only influence affective phenomena through physio-psychical phenomena. The psycho-physiological conditions can be brought into relation with several essential facts, one of which is relatively primitive, the arrest of certain tendencies, while the rest may in some cases be concomitant, and in others derived from the first.

We will consider the last-named characters later. For the moment we are concerned only with the first, the arrest of tendencies.

We will keep to the same example, assuming, of course, that the case is very marked. The arrested impulses are then numerous. Action, under the conditions which we have supposed, is generally accompanied by a certain hesitation : the shy man deliberates the whole way, and asks himself whether he shall go on to the end. His hesitation is sometimes so intense that he turns back when half-way, or even with his hand on the bell. In this case, all arrest of tendency ceases, and so do the affective features, unless others arise as a result of the arrest and lead to the accomplishment of the act (regret at lack of courtesy, unsatisfied curiosity, etc.). Moreover, if the shy man is not acquainted with the customs of society, he will not be too sure how to present himself; and should he be unacquainted with the people on whom he is calling, and ignorant of their character, manners, and habits, he will be equally uncertain as to the attitude which he should assume. And so it happens that many impulses which he feels to say or do various things are not completely rejected, but are inhibited and prevented from being translated into action. Moreover, tendencies to the free expression of normal character are checked, and speech-impulses are often inhibited to such an extent that the shy person does not know what to say, although ideas, that is tendencies to speech, may come to his mind in abundance. There is also a voluntary repression of instinctive movements which would tend to reveal bashfulness or embarrassment.

Suppose, on the other hand, that the habit has been formed. Suppose that tendencies are not arrested. The caller proceeds to a particular house, presents himself without difficulty, and utters the customary remarks ; everything is done without arrest of tendency, and also without the production of any affective phenomenon (at any rate in so far as these acts are concerned). Everything goes smoothly and sometimes even mechanically.

Whatever affective phenomenon we take, we can observe the same fact : the arrest of a tendency. From the most ordinary emotions to the highest and most complex feelings, we can always verify this law. Perhaps it is advisable, in order to avoid indefiniteness, to state clearly what must be understood by a *tendency* and by its arrest.

We have just seen that man may be regarded as a complex of phenomena, who to a certain extent tends to systematize himself and to systematize the world ; but it is not merely as a whole that he tends towards systematization. Every part of the physical or moral man has a tendency to organization on its own account, and organization of one part is frequently carried out at the expense of the organization of another. Thus in man we have a systematization or a juxtaposition of various small systems more or less bound together. We designate as a tendency the first part of the elements of one of these systems, those which, considered in relation to time, appear before the last and which consist in general of a certain activity of the nervous elements. If, for example, a fragment of bread, or any other substance I swallow, "goes the wrong way", and instead of entering the œsophagus gets into the larynx, we see that the tactile impressions of the foreign body, the centripetal impressions, the central act, and the motor impulses which cause the expulsion of the body by the contraction of the muscles, form an organized system, and converge towards a common goal ; we say, therefore, that the centripetal impressions and the central phenomena constitute a tendency to the appropriate muscular contraction. It is in the arrest of analogous tendencies that the affective phenomenon originates. In other words, by an arrested tendency I understand a more or less complicated reflex action which cannot terminate as it would if the organization of the phenomena were complete, if there were full harmony between the organism or its parts and their conditions of existence, if the system formed in the first place by man, and afterwards by man and the external world, were perfect. In hunger, in thirst, in all the organic needs which are manifested to consciousness by affective phenomena, we find arrested tendencies. Hunger is a general feeling of discomfort due to impoverishment of the blood. It is clear that this alone constitutes or entails a material arrest of tendencies. And if inanition is too prolonged, the arrest is all the more marked and the emotion also ; in this case, moreover, there is an arrest of the customary inclination to satisfy the appetite when it is felt. In all the other organic needs, such as the desire to micturate, to defecate, to emit semen, etc., we also find that the production of the affect is brought about by the arrest of a tendency, by an impediment to the systematization of certain psychical or physical elements. Sometimes, this arrest is specifically due to a greater systematization which is effected in the organism, as when we neglect to satisfy our hunger or thirst in order to finish some piece of work ; but this circumstance, which justifies the arrest of the lower impulse, does not always prevent us from being conscious of it.

Passing to the emotions caused by the exercise of our

B

senses, we find that they are all accompanied by an arrest of certain tendencies; a notable proof of this is supplied by the influence of habit, which, by rendering perception easier, lessens the affective phenomena. All the effects produced might perhaps be referred to this cause. Thus, when too bright a light dazzles the eyes and causes an unpleasant sensation, the habits of the eye are thwarted, and the established tendencies suffer arrest; similarly, a strident sound which grates upon the ear, a sharp body which tears the skin— all these suppress a whole series of organic habits of life.

At first glance, perhaps, it might seem that agreeable emotions, and in general all affects of a pleasurable character, are not referable to the same law. But, upon careful reflection, it will, I think, be found that here too, when the emotion is produced, it is due to the fact that a tendency encounters certain obstacles. For example, we find it pleasant to walk when we have remained still for a long while; but it is to be remarked that the exercise, even when it is accomplished with facility, is not performed without a certain effort, which is precisely what causes our pleasure. For once the effort has entirely disappeared, once we have walked for a good while, if we continue to walk at a more regular, more decided, more automatic pace, without the slightest effort, the movement is certainly facilitated; but the pleasure vanishes, and is replaced by automatism. It will be admitted that in the first moments of satisfaction, when a tendency to movement still remains to be satisfied, the accumulated psychical force is too considerable for the expenditure to be equal to the impulse, so that the latter still remains partially impeded. This view is supported by the facts; for, to keep to the same example, in the first moment of walking after a long rest, the energy which has been accumulated tends to expend itself not only in the movements which constitute walking but also in different and varied movements—leaping, gestures, shouting, etc. And the affective phenomenon lasts just as long as this superfluity of energy, that is to say, this arrested tendency continues. Pleasure and pain, then, imply a general condition common to both in so far as they are both affective states ; and similarly they would be found to have other common conditions, still more general, in so far as they were both considered, for example, in relation to the more general quality of being states of consciousness. Since we are not concerned here with the special psychology of affective phenomena, we need not inquire at the moment what special conditions make such phenomena pleasant or unpleasant.

If we ascend in the hierarchy of human needs and deal with desires of a higher order, we still find that they only give rise to affective phenomena when the tendency awakened undergoes inhibition. There, in my opinion, lies the explanation of the charm of ' forbidden fruit.' A prohibition is an obstacle, more or less formidable and real, which hinders the manifested tendency from attaining its end as easily as it might have done. Then, even when the tendency is satisfied, it suffers a check, which, according to its strength and the conditions which prevail at the time, is associated with agreeable or disagreeable emotions, such as fear, the peculiar pleasure of ' forbidden fruit ', the joy in surmounting obstacles, remorse, and the like ; but it is always accompanied by some emotion. We may recall the remark of the Spanish lady who, after indulging in some trivial pleasure, regretted that it had not been mortal sin to enjoy it. In other words, a little hindrance would have intensified the emotion. Everybody knows that a prohibition often increases the desire which it is intended to repress, even when it is obeyed, and if the contrary sometimes occurs, it is only because then, for some reason, the tendency is weakened or disappears. The cessation of the affective phenomena, in this case, is not due to the arrest of the tendency, but to its disappearance or enfeeblement, as we shall presently see more clearly.

It is unnecessary to insist on this point as regards a great many intellectual or moral tendencies. It has long been observed that feelings of moral satisfaction or remorse are blunted by habit, that is to say when the acts committed are not obstructed by the influence and functioning of physio - psychological processes antagonistic to the tendencies giving rise to the acts. The analysis of remorse especially has shown that it is produced by the awakening of certain tendencies occurring after their temporary enfeeblement. It is easy to see here an arrest in the awakening of higher tendencies. In fact, when the mind, returning to habits long formed and firmly rooted, re-discovers the trace of acts committed under the temporary influence of entirely opposite tendencies, a conflict is set up between the higher inclinations and the traces left by the lower impulses, in the shape of memories or incipient habits. The higher inclinations tend to systematize the mind, the imagination, and conduct in a certain way, and the process is arrested by what remains of the temporary influence of opposite tendencies; it is this check which, in the peculiar circumstances of its production, gives rise to the affective phenomena of remorse.

In another connection it has been said that there is more pleasure in seeking truth than in finding it, and that if we knew everything, nothing would remain but to finish with life, in order to avoid endless boredom. Without for the moment criticizing this proposition, I will confine myself to remarking that such part of it as may be true is an implicit recognition of the significance of arrest in the genesis of emotions.

I cannot examine in detail all the emotions and feelings, such as love, ambition, and fear, in order to discover and indicate in each the arrest of a tendency; I believe that the task would be more lengthy than useful, but I would indicate certain special points which may bear on the discussion.

To allow that a feeling or emotion is due to the arrest of a tendency, is to admit that every feeling, every emotion, in a word, every affective phenomenon, is accompanied by a tendency; that it does not exist absolutely and by itself, but is part of a system and belongs to a process whose perfect culmination would generally be a movement. This is not obvious, perhaps, at first sight; the corresponding tendency for such feelings as admiration, pure æsthetic emotion, etc., may not be immediately obvious. That certain feelings have an active side it is impossible to deny; that all feelings have an active side is difficult to affirm, and yet, in my opinion, there are strong reasons for admitting the truth of this proposition.

To begin with, there are a priori reasons in the principles of general psychology explained at the beginning of this volume. Indeed, if man is a totality of systems, receiving external impressions, systematizing them, and reacting in such a way as to introduce into himself and into the world a greater harmony in any particular point or in the whole, then all the phenomena that are exhibited in the apparatus which effects this adaptation in his nervous system have the direct or indirect result of exercising a greater or less influence upon his mode of reaction ; that is to say, it is a cause, a more or less essential condition, of the movements that compose the varied reactions of the human organism. But we can perhaps approach the question in a more exact and conclusive manner by direct observation.

Let us take the feeling which appears to be the most contemplative and the least active : admiration. It is easy to see that it does not occur without a tendency to behave in a certain way, as, for example, to be like the object of our admiration. This, in some cases, is obvious. To admire a hero, whether real or not, is to be disposed in some degree to act like him in analogous circumstances. If, when we are aware of feeling admiration, we imagine ourselves in different circumstances (supposing that we are not favourably placed for the imitation of the person we admire), we immediately bring out the tendency ; and this tendency sometimes betrays itself in rudimentary efforts towards action, and at least becomes conscious. When circumstances permit, and the tendency, although so far impeded that it gives birth to a phenomenon of the affective order, is yet free to terminate in action, it becomes still more evident and the action takes place. It is said that Seleucus, after hearing an account of the clemency of Augustus towards Cinna, was so overcome by admiration that he pardoned one of his adversaries who had been condemned to death. In the case of admiration for an individual, the tendency to action, though not always at first sight conscious, may thus be disclosed by appropriate reactions.

In other cases it is not so easy. Sometimes the tendency to act is less marked, because it is checked too early in its operation. What happens in us, for instance, when we admire a beautiful landscape? Let us consider this case. It is very evident that in the pleasure caused by the sight of the landscape there is something besides the delight of the eye, a delight which, by the way, is also accompanied by certain tendencies to particular movements. There is an intellectual pleasure due to some faint reminiscence of the agreeable impressions experienced on another occasion or occurring at the moment : the freshness of the air, awareness of temperature or season, visual or auditory sensations, etc. A confused and scarcely perceptible revival, it is true, but a real revival. In the absence of imagination, concrete or abstract, the landscape would cause no other emotion than that which would be produced by so many patches of colour, more or less harmoniously grouped. But these recollections, these images in the nascent state, are accompanied by an assemblage of tendencies — also in the nascent state and consequently almost imperceptible, to make movements which will cause us to enjoy those feelings again, or which are associated with them. Here, moreover, we can use a crucial experiment to disclose concealed tendencies. Suppose that the place which arouses our admiration is within our reach, that we can easily go there, that we are not tired—suppose, in short, an absence of everything that might check the full manifestation of impulses, should they be present, and we shall see those impulses end in movements ; admiration will give way to desire, desire to action. Hence, admiration is a tendency towards desire and consequently towards action, even in cases where the emotion appears to be essentially contemplative.

Pure æsthetic emotion may also be referred to the same law. It differs a little from the emotion we have just analysed, in that the tendencies are still less clear and can scarcely be displayed except by indirect methods. Æsthetic emotion, which belongs to the same class as moral emotion—if, indeed, the moral emotion be not a particular case of the æsthetic— consists in the particular impression which we experience when we have established in our minds the representation and comprehension of a work of art or an assemblage of any notably systematized objective phenomena ; or, again, when an external phenomenon which does not present this character of complexity and synthesis awakens in the mind an assemblage of systematized phenomena.[1] The particular characteristic of the æsthetic emotion is that the subject of admiration is considered in itself and for itself ; the emotion is produced by the correspondence among themselves of the various parts of the object causing the emotion

---

[1] In this connection, see my article on "l'Emotion esthétique" in the *Revue philosophique*, June, 1885.

or impression, not by the relationship of the object, considered as a whole, with other objects. The æsthetic emotion so understood may be regarded as due to the weak stimulation of a large number of tendencies. In this case the stimulation is too weak ever to terminate in action. It is even too faint to be recognized by the inner sense as a tendency to action, but we can easily see that it involves an awakening of sensations and ideas which in other circumstances obviously tend to produce actions. And it is precisely because the tendency is unable in this case to reach its customary goal, because it is absolutely inhibited as soon as produced, that the phenomena are considered by themselves, and not as means to a special end ; and that, as we have seen, is a characteristic of æsthetic emotion.

To return to the example cited above : if we think, on seeing the picture of a landscape, that it would be pleasant to walk in the place which it represents, we are not experiencing a pure æsthetic emotion. Here the tendency is not awakened consciously. The factors which produce it are certainly aroused in the mind, but they fail to combine in a manner similar to that which elicits the conscious tendency to action ; the active tendencies inherent in every psychical phenomenon are here arrested as soon as the phenomenon appears. This clearly differs from the admiration which we previously analysed only insofar as the active tendency in the present case is inhibited more quickly and completely. The æsthetic emotion is peculiar, therefore, in being due to a complex stimulation, highly systematized and arrested at the point where the tendency created by the stimulus gives rise to phenomena of sensation and intelligence.

I find confirmation of this theory in Spencer's remarks upon the Useful and the Beautiful in his *Essays*. According to Spencer, æsthetic emotion is frequently excited by objects which in former days were useful to our ancestors. Obviously this is easily explained by the theory which I have expounded. The sight and, in general, the sensory perception of those objects were formerly associated with a certain number of very frequently performed actions, and consequently tended to initiate certain systems of movements, so that actions at that epoch were often determined by the visual, tactile, and auditory sensations awakened by the objects in question. Nowadays, on the contrary, if the tendency does appear, thanks to heredity and to the physical structure we have acquired, or to the knowledge we possess of ancient customs, it is instantly checked by the various habits to which the conditions of our actual existence have given rise ; and as a rule it is not even consciously recognized as the starting-point of a particular system of determined actions. These, as we have seen, are the conditions of æsthetic emotion.[1]

By way of concluding the direct analysis of the general conditions of emotion, we may remark that when impulses of a certain strength are lacking, feelings are also absent. Probably all of us have noticed that the times when we are least impelled to action are those when we are most indifferent. This is generally explained by the supposition that feeling is the cause of action. I shall have occasion to return to this point later, but for the moment I will merely call attention to the fact that the sensitive and active faculties are generally affected at the same time.

I have spoken of strong impulses. We shall in fact see that the tendency to activity must have attained a certain strength before an affective phenomenon is produced ; and this is connected more directly with the second character of the cause of affects, viz. the multiplicity of the psychical phenomena which accompany

---

[1] This introduces a phenomenon analogous to those which Setchénoff has examined in his *Études psychologiques*. I would here call attention to the important part played by inhibition in Setchénoff's psychology. The idea of inhibition as the cause of desire was suggested by Bain in *The Emotions and the Will*.

them. Moreover, it is not only in normal states that the phenomenon just mentioned occurs, for we also find that in morbid conditions of the mind the absence of impulse coincides with the diminution of affective phenomena. For example, the following statement was made by a patient suffering from the nervous disease which Dr Krishaber called cerebro-cardiac neuropathy :

"My *affective faculties* were as much disordered as the others ; I became indifferent to my friends and my family ; only after an effort could I attend to my children when they were ill. . . .

"When I was not excited, I was silent, depressed, completely indifferent to everything. . . .

"Apart from fits of intense emotion, I was without will and without energy. The spirit of initiative was shattered within me."[1]

Finally, by indirect methods we can also throw light upon the part which inhibition of tendencies plays in the production of affective phenomena. This seems to have been established, for example, by the researches of physiologists upon the rise of the temperature of the nervous centres in activity and the rush of blood to the brain.

I transcribe an experiment by Schiff, cited by Herzen.[2] It is obvious that an experimental modification, arranged so as to cause a more active impulse and a corresponding emotion, is translated by an increase in the temperature of the brain, in other words, by a cerebral activity more considerable and less automatic, more complex and more inhibited.

"When everything was ready for the experiment, we offered the animal several times a little piece of paper with nothing in it. At first a slight deflection of the mirror was obtained, but it gradually diminished, and, after several consecutive repetitions, became almost *nil*.

[1] Krishaber, *De la névropathie cérébro-cardiaque*, Obs. II.
[2] Herzen, " Echauffement des centres nerveux par le fait de leur activité," *Revue philosophique*, 1877, I, 46.

A morsel of toasted bacon was then placed in the paper, which was again brought near to the muzzle of the still motionless animal. The nostrils of the dog visibly dilated, he smelt the paper, and at the same time a sudden deflection of five to eight degrees was observed on the galvanometer. The mirror did not immediately return to zero, but moved back one or two degrees, to deviate a second time two, three, or even four degrees; this return, followed by a fresh deviation, was frequently repeated a third time. During these oscillations, the animal still had the morsel of bacon under his nose. Sometimes in the course of these experiments there were movements of the head, but, unless they were excessive, they did not cause stronger or more rapid deflections of the mirror. With the more apathetic animals, which I chose deliberately for this class of observations, among such as were inclined to eat, the movements were restricted to those resulting from scent; and notwithstanding this, the deviation was so pronounced that it could not be confused with the oscillations produced by the mere presentation of the empty paper. When, instead of bacon, a small sponge soaked in creosote was put in the paper, the deflection increased, but never so much as when cooked bacon, cheese, or bones were offered, even in the case of animals which were still too ill to take solid food, and which afterwards refused to eat the very substances that had stimulated their sense of smell during the experiments." [1]

We find proofs of the increased flow of blood through the brain in the valuable experiments of Mosso, and in such observations as the following : " We were watching in complete silence the curve which the cerebral pulse was tracing upon the registering apparatus, the subject being a woman whose brain was in places exposed by a wound in the skull, when suddenly, and

---

[1] See also, upon the relations between emotion and the temperature of the brain : Hack Tuke, *Illustrations of the Influence of the Mind on the Body.*

without apparent cause, the pulsations became more frequent and the brain became dilated. . . . She told me afterwards that while absent-mindedly casting her eyes upon the cupboard opposite she had seen a skull among the books, which made her think of her malady and occasioned a terrible emotion."[1] A similar fact is attested by a friend of Mosso's, who was associated in his experiments. The basis of those experiments, as we know, is the decrease of blood in the body, especially in the arm, while the blood flows forcibly to the brain : "While he was standing before the registering apparatus, with his arms in two glass cylinders filled with water, Professor Ludwig entered. There was an immediate fall in the two points which indicated the volume of the arms, leaving on the paper a vertical black line about ten centimetres in length. This was the first time that I had seen so considerable a diminution in the volume of the hand and forearm under the influence of an apparently slight emotion."[2]

Thus far analysis has enabled us to recognize an arrest of tendencies in every affective phenomenon. We may now employ synthesis to give us the counter-proof and show that when a tendency is developed and suffers a check, it gives rise to emotions and feelings.

We have a valuable example of the birth of an emotion from the arrest of a tendency in the abnormal working of certain organic functions. For example, we breathe without experiencing any emotion so long as the reflex action which involves the lungs, the ribs, the diaphragm, etc., encounters no obstacle. No affective phenomenon is produced. If, on the contrary, we try to hold our breath, or if any obstruction impedes our movements, the arrested tendency gives rise to impressions of suffocation and pain. Purely organic functions are the occasion of emotive phenomena of this sort when they are interfered with. "The stomach, which usually gives us

[1] Mosso, *la Peur*, p. 49.
[2] *Ibid.*, p. 68.

very few sensations, may in a pathological condition cause us to be acutely conscious of the presence of food or foreign bodies."[1] Here the phenomenon is as clear as possible ; so long as the function is freely performed we are unconscious of it ; whenever it is hindered we experience an emotion. The phenomenon of arrest is especially well illustrated by painful emotions, but we have reason to believe that agreeable impressions are also due to the arrest of a motor impulse.

The stimulation provided by the genital organs when fully developed, and the multitude of emotions and feelings derived from them, furnish a good example of this psychological synthesis, which shows us the formation of a tendency and its arrest, with the resultant affective phenomena. Let us consider normal desire, occurring when the physiological conditions for its satisfaction have made their appearance. I am quite aware that this is not always the case, but the exceptions do not in any respect invalidate the law of arrest in the production of emotion. It may be, indeed, that certain brains are organized so as to experience sexual desire, not as a result of the stimulus proceeding from the sexual organs, but because of some other stimulus ; imagination, example, and heredity must play a part in this phenomenon, which is another case of emotion caused by inhibition. But we can afford to ignore these cases for the purpose in hand. There is no doubt that sexual desire is normally excited by a particular state of the organism, inducing an inclination to perform certain acts. The affective phenomena derived from the arrest of this tendency and from inability to satisfy it, either partially or completely, according to circumstances, have frequently been described. " The feeling of ennui at puberty ", says Esquirol, " is the result of a vague want, the nature of which is unknown to the person experiencing it. This need gives rise to restlessness, which induces melancholy, which, in its turn, leads to

---

[1] Kuss and Duval, *Cours de physiologie.*

listlessness."[1] Griesinger gives a description of the
pathological consequences of an excessive inhibition
of the impulse towards sexual intercourse. " It is not
uncommon, especially in women, for this circumstance
(the non-fulfilment of the genital functions) to have a
prominent share in causing insanity ; and in general,
it also gives a certain stamp to manias which break out
under the influence of other causes : the long-repressed
inclination is then made manifest, usually in the shape
of an erotic and sexual frenzy, sometimes merely ideal,
sometimes openly sensual."[2]

We shall note elsewhere, in connection with the
formation and organization of character, how certain
tendencies are formed by the combination and systematization of others.   For the moment, I will content
myself with calling attention to the fact and noting that
the law of arrest is further verified by this synthesis.
Thus the need to smoke may become very imperious,
once the act to which it leads has become a habit :
severe suffering may result if the impulse occasioned
by the habit be absolutely thwarted, and keen enjoyment if it be satisfied—not fully, but to a sufficient
extent. Nevertheless, the taste for tobacco is not inborn,
and, as a rule, the first time a man smokes the act is
not strictly occasioned by the desire for the particular
sensation it produces, since as yet he knows nothing of
it.   Moreover, the performance is not always pleasant
at the first attempt ; it is manifest, therefore, that the
act and the impulse, as I shall describe later on, tend
to become a habit and give rise to a persistent tendency,
and that the beginnings of the tendency are the cause,
and not the consequence, of the affects which are produced. Hence we see that pleasure or pain, and affective
phenomena in general, should not be considered as
a cause of the act; but the tendency to action really
precedes and occasions the emotive phenomena.   The

[1] Esquirol, *Maladies mentales*, I, p. 553.

[2] Griesinger, *Traité des maladies mentales*, p. 236.

recognition of such a law led Pascal to advise religious exercises as a means of awakening belief. It is a fact that without the stimulus of affective phenomena we may form certain habits whose development and arrest subsequently produce affective phenomena which seem to be the cause of the tendency. Thus it sometimes happens that we have difficulty in breaking trivial habits carelessly formed, which never produced well-defined emotions when they were satisfied, but which when interfered with or discontinued cause discomfort and sometimes make such a blank in our lives that we cannot give them up. In fact, other things being equal, an action is easier to execute the more often it has been performed, and the tendency to accomplish it becomes stronger and is more easily and frequently aroused. There are various possibilities : either the tendency is completely satisfied, in which case the habit becomes mechanical, almost unconscious, and changes into instinct ; or it is sufficiently satisfied, and the arrest is enough to cause some degree of desire and some degree of pleasure upon satisfaction ; or, again, the impulse becomes too strong, the means of satisfying it are inadequate, the arrest is more marked, and then we have affects of another kind, grief, regret, etc., until the tendency is satisfied or removed—until there is no further check, or no more inclination.

The last case, where the tendency increases more rapidly than the means of satisfying it, will probably cover the following instance cited by M. Legrand du Saulle, after Trélat : " Mme de X. belonged to a wealthy family of high traditions. Her mother, notwithstanding her riches, took pains to train her in rigid principles and modest habits. The two spent a great part of the year in the country, where this girl showed herself to be of an easy disposition and very simple tastes. She amused herself by rearing birds in an aviary and looking after her collection of butterflies. No other pleasure was known to her before she reached the age of twenty-

two, the time of her marriage. But no sooner had she
experienced sexual relations than insatiable libidinous
appetites began to develop, and these found only too
many occasions for their exhibition."[1] M. Griesinger
also mentions a number of facts which show how tendency and stimulation have priority over feeling. "In
the male sex, disturbances of the genital functions—
known as involuntary seminal discharge, etc.—are of
considerable importance. Such anomalies, in which,
of course, the loss of seminal fluid is rarely the principal
fact, frequently depend, as Lallemand demonstrated,
upon local affections of the urethral mucous membrane,
the seminal vesicles, etc. ; in other cases they originate
especially in the nervous system ; usually they are preceded by a fairly long period of sexual hyper-activity
(excessive discharges) which is less the cause of these
anomalies than a symptom of the existence of considerable irritation of the parts ; once established, these
anomalies are marked by a more or less complete sup-
pression of sexual desire, by a great diminution of
erection, and by impotence, associated with all possible
disorders of sensibility and of morale, which sometimes amount to hysteria in the man and at other times
produce a condition of profound hypochondria."[2]

Moreover it is immaterial whether impulses to movement appear as the consequence of an external stimulus
or whether they proceed from within ; they may, in
appearance at least, be purely cerebral in character.
Such, for example, are the impulses of certain neuro-
paths and lunatics. Here, again, the affective phenomena appear to be preceded by the impulse which gives
them birth, and to become clearer and stronger according
as the impulse increases. " These lamentable impulses ",
remarks Esquirol, speaking of certain tendencies to
murder, "are not provoked by hatred or anger, as in

---

[1] Legrand du Saulle, Appendix on Nymphomaniacs in *Les Hystériques*,
pp. 599-600.
[2] Griesinger, *Op. cit.*, p. 237.

raving maniacs ; they are spontaneous, fleeting, foreign, even in habitual delirium. . . . Sometimes homicidal monomaniacs are torn by an internal struggle between the impulse to murder and the feelings and motives which cause repulsion from it ; the violence of the struggle is proportionate to the power of the impulse and the degree of intelligence and sensibility retained. That is so true that frequently the insane, whatever the character of their delirium, have inclinations towards murder, but these inclinations have no violence ; in others the wish to kill is powerful and frequently renewed, and the patient fights against it. With some, the impulse is more energetic, it sets up an external struggle which perturbs and worries the patient and throws him into terrible distress ; lastly, in a few cases, the impulse is so violent and instantaneous that there is no struggle and the deed follows immediately." [1]

Finally, psychological experiment has shown that a person in a state of induced somnambulism can be made to perform some pre - arranged action, even a fairly long while after his awaking. Here a tendency is directly created without the intervention of any sensation whatever, and the facts prove that this tendency, when repressed, is accompanied by affective phenomena. To quote Richet : " I say to V. ' Fondle this dog '. At once she proceeds to caress it. If the dog tries to shun her embrace, V. runs after him, follows him in all his movements, and if he goes out of the room tries to catch him again. If a chair or bench is placed in her way, she overturns the obstacle, or, if unsuccessful, becomes exasperated and pushes it away angrily. . . If I tell A. to dress herself and go out, she at once goes to get the things needed for her toilet: at first she reflects, then, after due consideration, she goes with her eyes closed to seek the object in its customary place. Meditation upon the act is slow, but the act itself is accomplished with extraordinary animation. If a fasten-

---

[1] Esquirol, *Op. cit.*, II, p. 104.

C

ing, a string, or any other obstacle, offers some resistance, A. becomes fretful and irritable, and angrily
throws aside everything that checks her purpose." [1]

There is no need, I think, to continue further this
demonstration of the phenomenon of arrest as a condition
necessary to the production of affective phenomena.
But, though every affect is produced by an arrest of
tendencies, not every arrest of tendencies causes an
affective phenomenon. We shall see in the following
chapters, when we come to study other conditions of
the production of affects, that the arrest of a tendency
may be accompanied simply by an intellectual phenomenon or by no phenomenon of consciousness whatever. The inquiry into the other conditions for the
appearance of emotions and feelings will enable us to
formulate the law of arrest with more precision and to
indicate the character of this arrest both in general and
in the particular case in which it is connected with the
production of an affect.

II. *The multiplicity of the phenomena*

That a multiplicity of nervous and conscious phenomena should constitute one of the principal characteristics of the production of an emotion might to some
extent be deduced a priori from the first characteristic
which we recognized in connection with affective
phenomena. In fact, if the production of an emotion
be always accompanied by the arrest of a tendency,
above all if that tendency is sufficiently strong—a
condition which, relatively at least, is necessary—the
nervous energy absorbed by the tendency must be
expended in the production of other purely nervous
or neuro-psychic phenomena, and this will obviously
be a constant characteristic of emotion. This explanation cannot, however, be absolutely generalized. There
are phenomena of inhibition, for example, to which

[1] Ch. Richet, *L'Homme et l'intelligence,* pp. 188-189 (1884).

the preceding formula is only indirectly applicable, and the various modes of nervous action are not yet sufficiently well-known to enable psychology to derive all the profit possible from physiological discoveries. Furthermore, whatever the immediate cause and the physiological nature of nervous disturbances, direct and indirect observation and all the methods of investigation we possess for recognizing the existence of nervous and psychical phenomena show us a remarkable multiplicity of factors accompanying the appearance of a phenomenon of the affective order. These concomitant phenomena may be of various kinds ; they can be physical or psychical, and the latter may be either intellectual or affective.

1. The physical phenomena accompanying emotions are familiar to most people, and have been studied under the name of " the expression of the emotions ". I need only mention the works of Darwin, Spencer, Dumont, and Mantegazza, to show the importance of the subject. It is not in accordance with the plan of the present inquiry to make a special study of the expression of the emotions. We have only to recall that the movements which constitute that expression appear, *other things being equal*, to increase according as the emotion itself increases ; that is to say, according as the impulse is stronger and the arrest more marked. We observe further that the expression of the emotions generally involves the arrest of the tendency that engenders them. Certain movements, indeed, are simply the outline of the gestures which the general systematization of the organism would command. The motion of recoil, for instance, which is caused by a sensation of horror, is the outline or initiation of a system of actions tending to withdraw the organism from causes which tend to destroy it. What is menaced in idea, or, in other words, feebly arrested, is here our ordinary habit of mind and imagination, and the sum of the tendencies which make up our personality ; this arrest and the multiplicity of phenomena deriving

from it, among which there is generally a pronounced movement of recoil, while the hands will be stretched out as if to avert danger, give rise to an affective phenomenon. At other times the movements seem to have no logical connection with the cause of the emotion ; that is, they do not form part of a system, but result from a non-systematized diffusion of the nervous energy aroused. In this class of phenomena we must include the convulsive movements which accompany grief or joy, and particularly the phenomena of laughter. Léon Dumont and Herbert Spencer have both established the general fact that the movements of laughter are produced by a nervous stimulation which we do not find in the nervous phenomena accompanying ideas or feelings. Their theories, though they differ in detail, agree as to this general fact, which is all that concerns us at the moment. Here, no doubt, should also be included the cases in which a nervous stimulation gives rise to a feeling, and then to a convulsion and an epileptic fit. Habit plays a part in the causation of the phenomenon, and it seems as though, in some instances and with certain persons, the nervous stimulation, arrested and engendering an emotion of a special kind, is transformed into an epileptic fit, just as in other persons and in other circumstances it is manifested by a special gesture, peculiar to the individual or common to a large number of people. " The readiness with which attacks (of epilepsy) recur ", observes Esquirol, " seems to show that after the organism has once been so affected the nervous system retains a special disposition, which the slightest cause brings into action, inducing further paroxysms. . . A woman in acute grief becomes an epileptic ; the slightest trouble provokes fresh attacks. A child is scared by a dog and becomes epileptic ; he has a fit every time he hears a dog bark. . . Another becomes epileptic after an outburst of passion ; the slightest opposition brings on fits." [1]

----

[1] Esquirol, *Op. cit.*, Vol. I, pp. 296-297.

2. Besides movement, there are other phenomena which likewise accompany the production of affects; these are the functional phenomena exhibited by the organs of vegetative life. Bain, Maudsley, and Claude Bernard have made a study of this subject. I shall make but a brief reference to them here, and that merely in order to show how many and diverse are the factors which go to the making of the conditions of emotion. "Emotion", remarks Maudsley, "will often increase, lessen, or alter a secretion, bidding the tears flow, perverting the bile, making the tongue cleave to the roof of the mouth ; and it may be questioned whether there is a single act of nutrition which emotion may not affect, inspiring it with energy or infecting it with feebleness, according to its pleasant or painful nature." [1]

According to Bain, the organic effects of emotion manifest themselves chiefly in the lachrymal gland, the sexual and digestive organs, the skin, the heart, the lungs, and the mammary glands. Every one knows that certain keen emotions, joy, enthusiasm, tenderness, and especially suffering, may increase the secretion of tears until weeping is occasioned ; depressing passions take away the appetite and disturb the functioning of the stomach, the liver, and the intestines. Fear may bring about paralysis of the nerves of the intestines, and especially of the vaso-motor nerves, thus giving rise to an abundance of liquid products in the intestinal duct. Further noteworthy facts, attested by various authorities, arc the feeling of suffocation which is produced in the pharynx during paroxysms of intense pain, and changes in perspiration : the secretion of perspiration is dependent upon the influence of the nervous system, and fear or a depressing emotion will bring on cold sweats. The movements of the heart, as we know, are powerfully influenced by feelings and emotions through the medium of the pneumo-gastric nerve. Modifications of respiration, sobbing, blushing due to shame and

[1] Maudsley, *The Physiology of Mind*, p. 385.

anger, are likewise phenomena upon which we need not dwell. The numerous and ill-co-ordinated physiological phenomena which accompany the affect supply us with one of its most marked characteristics. In purely intellectual activity this important train of physiological facts is not observable ; not that they are entirely wanting, but they are far less numerous and, above all, not nearly so obvious.

3. Lastly, psychical phenomena are no less abundant than the others. With emotion we always find a long sequence of ideas and feelings, sometimes logical and sometimes incoherent, which arise and assail the mind. When a somewhat pronounced tendency is inhibited, or at least impeded to a sufficient extent, this train of psychical phenomena is scarcely ever absent. Consider the case of a mistake about a rendezvous. One person is waiting for another, and the time of the appointment passes without any sign of him. Here there is evidently an arrest of tendencies which of course vary according to the object of the meeting. But if we presume that it is a matter of importance, a business or a love affair, the arrested tendencies will give rise to a host of phenomena which will vary according to the case. The imagination is set going, and accessory feelings are awakened ; conjectures, quite probable at first and afterwards highly improbable, will presently be made, if the person is one of those in whom associations are easily formed. A nervous woman, whose husband or child does not return punctually for dinner, readily fancies that he has been robbed, murdered, or run over; and these ideas, by bringing about the arrest of fresh tendencies or by accentuating that arrest, yield new emotions and a further series of ideas. Here is a case in point : a child four or five years old was accustomed to see his mother come to his bedside every morning and stay with him. One morning he was left alone longer than usual. Boredom to begin with, then impatience, then dread, followed this arrest of tendencies. Emotion found

physical expression in cries ; the child called his mother, then his nurse, then a neighbour, but nobody heard him ; it also took the form of movements, tears, etc. Psychically the phenomena were not less numerous ; he reflected upon the causes which might explain the delay ; he passed from one to another, and eventually imagined that his parents had perhaps gone away or even that they had changed their house and temporarily forgotten him. " A child ", he thought, " may be forgotten." Notice that his personal experience in no wise entitled him to have ideas such as these and that he did not himself take them very seriously, but under compulsion his imagination worked, and the intellectual and affective phenomena were multiplied.

When tendencies whose normal functioning occasions no affective or even conscious phenomenon are impeded, we have seen that their arrest is accompanied by emotions or feelings. In this case, moreover, it is easy to observe that the production of the feeling is always associated with the activation of a relatively larger number of psychical elements. Thus breathing, which in the normal state is a comparatively simple process, becomes highly complicated from the psychological aspect when it is checked, and gives rise to particular emotions. The very birth of these emotions is a complication ; besides, many ideas and images appear—ideas created in order to shake off the oppression, and images generated by them. The process is the same whatever the tendency checked and the emotion exhibited. Thirst, hunger, love and hatred, when the feeling is sufficiently strong, are accompanied by a great number of ideas and images, either coherent and systematized, as when passion and desire suggest to men the means of satisfying them and those means are appropriate ; or less coherent, and even wholly disconnected, in the case of ideas and images awakened, perhaps, simply by resemblance and contiguity, or by some association whose nature can scarcely be ascertained.

The first characteristic is probably the most note-worthy, although it is not the most frequent, even in ordinary life. But we are in the habit of believing that those almost completely systematized associations which constitute reason play a much more important part in human life than they actually do. Besides, we often regard reasoning as in some way more natural than other processes and quite different from them. I should also urge, were this the appropriate place, that system-atized association has been too much neglected by the majority of psychologists of the empirical school, for it is important to discover whether systematized associa-tion can be referred to association by contiguity and similarity, or whether, on the contrary, associations by contiguity and similarity cannot be referred to and ex-plained by systematized association. It will suffice at this point to deal with the part played by the various modes of association in the production of feeling.

If, therefore, adopting this point of view, we examine the numerous phenomena exhibited in the birth of an emotion, we shall find that they are as a rule some-what ill-systematized, either among themselves or in relation to the whole organism. A great many of the processes of organic life induced by a strong emotion appear to have no utility; and, in a general way, the more notable their affective character, the more in-harmonious will be the manifestations of the emotion. Thus a man whose anger is moderate still finds good arguments with which to confront his opponent, and sensible reproaches to bring against him. But if his anger becomes uncontrollable the chances are that he will only be able to bring out ridiculous phrases, in-vective, and meaningless oaths, or scarcely articulate exclamations. I will not labour the point, for it is common knowledge that in extreme emotions and passions one 'loses one's head'. On the view here taken, this means that the arrest of an exceedingly powerful impulse is accompanied by the production of a mass of badly systematized psychical phenomena. We may recall in this connection the influence of affective phenomena on the production of insanity, which is nothing other than a loss of harmony among the psycho-organic phenomena themselves, or in relation to the rest of the organism and the environment. "Among the moral causes" (of madness), says Griesinger,[1] "it is above all necessary to recognize the passions and emotions, for it is an undoubted fact that an exaggerated mental struggle alone, without a concomitant emotion or other important cause (any excess, as when insomnia is promoted by the use of stimulants) very rarely occasions madness. It is quite otherwise with strong or persistent emotions, and, in particular, with painful feelings of loss, etc., and depressing emotions; though it is extremely rare for immoderate joy alone to cause lunacy, if indeed it ever happens." Consequently, it is scarcely possible to be 'mad with joy', as the saying goes. Nevertheless the expression clearly denotes the disturbance of one of the conditions of emotion, and if the disturbance attendant upon joy is less profound than that which is occasioned by grief, the circumstance is by no means inexplicable : painful emotions are peculiar in that they tend to introduce ideas, feelings, and habits entirely at variance with the existing organization. No doubt, as Maudsley also remarks, if man could attain the power to moderate or regulate the affective or emotional element of his nature, the sum of insanity in the world would be considerably diminished; he would, in fact, be freed from the burden of the so-called moral causes of that malady. Very rarely, if ever, will insanity result from excess of intellectual activity; "it is when intellectual activity is accompanied with great emotional agitation that it is most enervating—when the mind is the theatre of great passions that its energy is soonest exhausted."[2]

---

[1] Griesinger, *Op. cit.*, p. 197.
[2] Maudsley, *The Physiology and Pathology of the Mind*, p. 245 (1867).

The experiments of physiologists have brought to light the law of the reflex phenomena of the spinal cord ; a stimulus applied to a frog's foot, for example, produces a reaction in the foot which felt the stimulus ; if the stimulation becomes stronger, the reaction is exhibited by a movement of both feet ; should it be yet further augmented, all four limbs move. As the stimulation increases, therefore, it is gradually diffused throughout the nervous system. Psychology yields facts of the same order, and some of these have been studied and offer confirmation of an analogous law. If an impulse be arrested or hindered, and the stimulus, whether coming directly or indirectly from outside, be very strong, we observe that the nervous energy at first expends itself in systematized impressions which association makes more readily accessible : but if the impulse increases, more distant associations occur. The stimulation becomes more general. It awakens systems of thoughts and impressions that are less directly connected with the cause of the impression, and even the associated movements become less and less systematized and resemble convulsions.

Here, as before, we can introduce a sort of counter-proof and show how, when the phenomena which we have just mentioned begin to disappear, the affect vanishes also, and vice versa. The method of difference, like the method of agreement, leads to this conclusion —that in the production of an affect a great number of psychical elements are roused. As before, we have a verification of the law in the effects of habit. For example, when something that once profoundly moved us happens to be repeated, if the emotion diminishes we also observe a diminution in the number of processes aroused by a kind of psychical reflex. If a joke which once made us laugh be repeated after a certain interval, it will arouse only a moderate degree of amusement ; if we hear it again, it leaves us cold, and our muscles do not stir ; neither emotion nor idea is evoked. As an illustration of arrest, I referred above to the first visit of a nervous man to people whom he does not know. I might have chosen it also to show the multitude of images, ideas, reflections, and even feelings which arise in the mind when an affective phenomenon is produced. Suppose that the habit is formed, and that the affect disappears ; the whole accompanying train disappears with it. There are no more preoccupations, no more reflections, comments, preparatory mental conversations and subjective sketches of gestures and greetings. Conversely, when phenomena multiply, we witness the birth of an emotion. This is what happens, for instance, when we are thinking over something and discover hitherto unperceived relations with other facts of which we suddenly become conscious. This process, which in the first place was purely intellectual, suddenly gives rise to affective phenomena, and just as we have recently seen the affective phenomenon gives way to a purely intellectual and almost automatic phenomenon, according to the decrease in the number of psychical elements, so we here observe a purely intellectual phenomenon being replaced by an emotion, when the number of psychical elements increases.

I mentioned above that the fact of arrest is not peculiar to affects. Indeed, an idea, a representation, a phenomenon which is simply intellectual, is also the result of the arrest of a tendency. Nor is multiplicity of phenomena absolutely peculiar to the production of affects. It is easy to see that an intellectual phenomenon, an idea, is accompanied by the production of a certain number of associated facts ; even attention, when it is focussed on one idea, is accompanied by a certain stimulation of the motor centres ; moreover, an intellectual matter generally suggests others connected with it. Yet this process is not quite the same in emotion and ideation. It is more systematized in the latter, more vivid and more confused in the former. When we think, ideas are usually awakened with a view to an end, whether we are following an argument, seeking out a cause, or deducing from an occurrence all its consequences. And in a general way, when we use our intellect, our reason, it is obvious that the phenomena are much better co-ordinated than when they are occasioned by that arrest of tendencies which produces an emotion. Emotion and feelings are a sort of disturbance of the organism, and even if we admit with Maudsley that it is the same on the whole with all our conscious processes (which I regard as highly probable), it must be agreed that the disturbance is much less pronounced where the intellect is concerned than in the case of feeling.

If we regard the subject from the point of view of general psychology, and if we accept the definition of tendency which I gave at the beginning of this work, every psychical event appears to us as a tendency, and every conscious process as the result of the arrest of a tendency. Indeed, we see that consciousness diminishes as the tendency encounters fewer and fewer obstacles. Purely reflex actions (those to which the name is generally applied) are the easiest, simplest and least conscious; they seem, in fact, to be totally unconscious. Just as the nervous system of man might be considered as an apparatus designed to receive diverse impressions and, by appropriate reactions, to put the various parts of the organism and the environment into a fairly advanced state of systematization, by the modification either of the organization or the environment, so every impression, every nervous stimulation, every psychical process, should be regarded as a tendency to bring about, prepare, or facilitate, movements of a diverse nature. All that we know about the physiological conditions of consciousness; the flow of the blood, the rise in temperature, the duration of the process, and the wear and tear of nerve tissue, entitles us to believe that consciousness is produced either when these tendencies have not been sufficiently satisfied to facilitate the path of excitation in the right degree or when some other condition (for instance the complexity and number of the systems of psychical elements brought into play, the intervention of other tendencies, and the ensuing conflict), causes an obstacle. In such cases the tendency to act cannot easily and immediately realize itself and so becomes manifest in a conscious process.

Commonplace events enable us to understand this phenomenon without difficulty. When we perform any action mechanically, and something interrupts this almost automatic movement, we suddenly become conscious of the thing we are doing. We do not always see this, but by examination of a few cases we shall be able to find the causes which sometimes allow the state of unconsciousness to persist, sometimes give rise to an intellectual event and sometimes, finally, occasion the appearance of an affect. We shall then have completed our account of the general cause of affective phenomena.

III. *Power and persistence of the impulse, sudden appearance and relative lack of co-ordination of phenomena. Tendency to encroach upon the whole field of consciousness*

We have recognized two principal characteristics in the production of emotions : the arrest of tendencies and the multiplicity of phenomena. But at the same time we saw that these two characteristics are insufficient to explain completely the birth of affective phenomena. We must, therefore, specify fully the conditions such phenomena should present. We have already had a glimpse of these special characteristics, but it is essential to examine them more closely. They are the strength and persistence of the inhibited impulse, the relatively sudden appearance and relative lack of co-ordination of the phenomena, and the tendency to invade the whole field of consciousness. These characteristics are secondary in the sense that they will not always be present at the same time in the production of emotions ; but they are essential, in that if none of them is present there is no affective but only an intellectual phenomenon. On the other hand, the first two characteristics which we considered are indispensable, although they are not sufficient alone.

1. *The power and persistence of the arrested tendency.* When an arrested tendency is not very strong, it is unusual for its inhibition to give rise to affective phenomena. It is rarely difficult to give up a recently adopted habit, because by simply omitting to perform the action we not only check the inclination but also cause it to disappear. Indirect means, therefore, are sometimes useful for preventing a child or grown person from doing something which ought not to be done. Very often we succeed better by attracting their attention to something else, by directing their thoughts from the forbidden act, than by running directly counter to their wishes. For in the first case the check of the tendency does not, as in the second, give rise to affects, since the tendency is not arrested but suppressed. Nor does it call forth, as in the case of the sudden arrest of a persistent impulse, the whole series of secondary phenomena and psychical reflexes. If we build a wall in the bed of a river, it will overflow its banks into the fields beyond, but if we draw off the water into a canal, there is neither an abrupt check nor an inundation. The psychical process is almost analogous to this.

The persistence of an arrested impulse, however, is not alone sufficient to produce an emotion : the impulse must also have a certain intensity. When this condition is fulfilled we see the affect arising and becoming more and more pronounced according as the persistent and arrested impulse becomes stronger. For example, without experiencing any emotion we can easily resist the vague idea of some action which may occur to us and which persists for some time ; but if the notion

becomes increasingly insistent, as is the case, for
instance, when it is the thought of an act satisfying an
organic requirement, a moment will arrive when the
arrest and the persistence of the impression must cause
an emotion or a feeling. Hunger, which at the outset
is hardly noticeable, and seems to be first a scarcely
conscious tendency and then a simple idea, gradually
becomes a very violent affect. Here is a case, taken
from Maudsley, which shows clearly how the persistence
of a tendency and its arrest are not always enough, but
how the intensifying of an impulse readily leads to an
affective phenomenon ; and again, how the latter, with
the physical and psychical phenomena inseparable from
it, may, in the conditions I shall indicate, take the place
of an almost purely intellectual phenomenon :

" Not long ago I was consulted by a man of fifty, with
enormous muscles and of great physical strength, who
had led an energetic life and in the course of his career
had visited nearly all parts of the world, but who for
several years had been without any active occupation.
He was possessed by an impulse to murder, and lived
in unceasing anguish. The obsession was continual,
and sometimes so intense that he was obliged to separate
himself from his relations for fear he should murder
them : he wandered from hotel to hotel. The impulse
varied considerably in intensity, but it never entirely
disappeared. When least strong, it was only an idea
constantly occupying his mind, but he was without
positive inclination to put it into execution ; a homicidal
notion rather than a homicidal impulse. From time to
time it became much more violent and reached a paroxysm.
It lasted only a short time, but while it lasted the blood
went to his head, which was oppressed by a sensation
of fullness and disturbance, his whole body was bathed in
a profuse perspiration and he trembled violently ; this
was accompanied by a terrible feeling of despair. The
crisis ended in a deluge of tears, followed by profound
exhaustion. These attacks often came on in the night,

when he would leap from his bed in a state of mortal terror shivering with such violence that the room shook : at these times sweat streamed from his body."

2. *The sudden appearance and relative lack of co-ordination of the phenomena.* There are general reasons for believing that affective phenomena are due to the imperfect functioning of the mind. The arrest of tendencies and the multiplicity of phenomena are signs of a lack of co-ordination and systematization. Experience has likewise shown us the peculiar characteristic of absence of co-ordination in those secondary phenomena which are produced, through a sort of reflex mechanism, by the arrest of a tendency. Yet this lack of co-ordination is not always very marked, and an emotion is frequently produced after a co-ordination between different phenomena has been established in the mind. This is the case, for example, with intellectual emotions. The lack of systematization is only manifest in the slight difficulty with which new ideas obtrude themselves, and in the often almost imperceptible resistance of old mental habits. But in this case another factor is frequently introduced which makes up for the first and produces an affect : that is, the abrupt appearance of phenomena. If our ideas change gradually, we are scarcely affected. If, on the contrary, we pass suddenly from one belief to another, the moment of change is marked by the very noticeable production of feelings and emotions. The weakness of the resistance put up by pre-existing mental habits is made up for by the speed with which they have to disappear, and the phenomenon of arrest, with all its consequences, may be sufficiently marked for an emotion to be felt.

At other times emotion is caused by the fact that if new combinations are set up in the mind, old combinations, still closely associated with a great number of tendencies and habits, are obliged to make room for them, with the result that the mind is considerably disorganized. This state of relative dissolution, except when extremely slow, always has an emotional counterpart, more or less intense. A famous instance of this peculiar condition is to be found in Jouffroy's account of the night when he definitely broke away from Catholicism : "In vain I clung to these last beliefs, as a castaway to the remnants of his ship ; in vain, terrified by the unknown void into which I was about to drift, I turned back with them, for the last time, to my childhood, my family, my country, to everything I held dear and holy: but the relentless current of thought was too strong ; relations, family, memories, beliefs—I was forced to abandon all ; the inquiry went on, more insistent and ruthless as the end approached, and it only ceased when that was reached. I knew then that the whole structure of my being was shattered to its very foundations.

"It was a terrible moment; and when towards the morning I threw myself exhausted upon my bed, I seemed to feel that my first life, so full and so happy, was dead, and that before me another was opening, sombre and desolate, in which henceforth I should live alone—alone with the fatal thought which had sent me into banishment, and which I was tempted to curse. The days that followed this discovery were the saddest of my life."[1]

So again we see these two characteristics, relative lack of co-ordination and the sudden appearance of phenomena, supplementing one another up to a certain point, as the persistence and intensity of the impulse were also seen to do. Furthermore, these different characteristics are not always disjoined : they may combine among themselves ; we find that very strong tendencies may persist for a very long time, and sometimes appear in an abrupt fashion. In the same way, the inco-ordination of phenomena may be greatly prolonged. The characteristics which we are at present studying may supplement and replace each other, but

---

[1] Jouffroy, *Nouveaux mélanges philosophiques*, p. 84.

D

they can also occur together and co-operate in the production of the same effect.

3. *The tendency to encroach upon the whole field of consciousness.* Here again is a characteristic which is not absolutely restricted to affective phenomena, although it appears to me to be frequently and intimately connected with them. It must be observed that this is not a necessary condition of an emotion or a feeling. Indeed, one may very well be under the impress of some emotion or feeling and yet be occupied with something other than its object; while, on the other hand, an idea, a purely intellectual phenomenon, may entirely absorb our attention. Nevertheless, this case may be regarded as doubtful; for extreme concentration is usually accompanied, so far as I am able to judge, by a kind of emotion, so that perhaps it may be viewed as a phenomenon of the affective order. When we are absorbed in any investigation, in any piece of work of an intellectual character, I believe that rarely, if ever, do we not experience some feeling of pleasure followed by fatigue, impatience or content. But in any case, as a general rule, a fairly keen emotion tends to engross us entirely and to occupy our whole mind. I need not insist upon this very common phenomenon, which is doubtless explained by the laws of association and selection.

The various characteristics which we have considered in isolation are to be seen active together and giving rise (according as they do or do not happen to be associated with the arrest of tendencies and the multiplicity of phenomena) to unconscious processes, or else to phenomena of the intellectual order, or finally, to emotions or feelings.

Thus, for example, if we are talking as we walk along, and the conversation becomes very interesting or animated, we stop, and walking is interrupted. Here we have an arrest of the impulse to motion, which is accompanied neither by feeling nor even by definite

consciousness. How does this come about? Walking
is a reflex action, and its stimulus is largely the
impression made by the ground upon the soles of the
feet—as observation of certain diseases has proved.
Now so long as one is walking, this excitation and the
tendency to movement persist; hence when the walking
stops, the tendency is also arrested. The conditions in
which this arrest is produced are the following: 1, the
impulse to walk is very weak, and sometimes is
gratified only because it encounters no obstacle; 2, the
impulse is not checked by any direct obstacle, but by
some other psycho-physiological process which has
remained independent of it for a while, but which now
absorbs all the psychical energy, including that which
was needed to put the walking impulse into action;
3, the tendency to walk is not merely hindered, but, for
the moment, almost suppressed—at all events no
conscious phenomenon relating to it is produced.

Now let us examine a case in which the arrest of a
tendency occasions conscious happenings.

When we are extremely absorbed by any occupation,
we finish by entirely losing all clear consciousness of
what we are doing; in this case, an interruption, which
forces us out of our abstraction, gives us or restores
to us that consciousness. Thus, if I am writing and
absorbed by my work, from time to time I shall make
use of the ink in my inkstand and preserve only a
very vague consciousness of the action, if indeed I am
sensible of it at all: but if my inkpot is empty, or if
something checks the almost unconscious impulse
to move my hand in its direction, when my pen begins
to form the letters badly I recover a distinct consciousness of the impulse, of my need, and of the
circumstances in which the impulse and the need become
manifest. Then representations and ideas occur—intellectual phenomena. If we analyse the circumstances of
this inhibition, we find that they are as follows: 1, the
impulse to write and to make all the movements which

pertain to that action encounters a direct impediment; it is not arrested because the psychical energy is summoned elsewhere, as would happen and does happen whenever a more intense concentration upon the subject of my reflections stays my pen. The impulse persists, and only awaits the disappearance of obstacles which have hindered it before expressing itself again in action ; 2, the new psychical phenomena which follow the impulse are related to that impulse. They are, specifically, images of ink, pen, paper, etc., ideas of the relations of these different objects to one another, representations of the gestures I must perform in order to procure ink, and tendencies towards the appropriate movements. These things are neither very numerous nor very complex, and they are fairly well systematized; 3, the accompanying psychical conditions, reflections upon the subject I am writing about, the pursuit of ideas, etc., are not wholly interrupted, and do not escape completely from the field of consciousness.

Let us next take a case in which an affective phenomenon is involved instead of an unconscious process or an intellectual phenomenon, noting the peculiarities exhibited at the same time. If, for instance, believing that he is accosting an intimate friend whom he has not seen for a long while, an effusive man throws himself with open arms on a stranger, the arrest of various tendencies which arise at the moment (gestures, words, etc.) is translated in this case into a feeling of confusion and regret. At the same time his imagination begins to work and vividly presents to him either the absurdity or the humour of the occurrence ; and if he is at all impressionable, if, that is to say, he is apt to experience for a moment feelings of great intensity, he will forget almost everything which is not more or less directly connected with what is happening to him ; his attention will be entirely engaged by the thoughts, images, and affective states which result from the arrest of these tendencies. Here then we find : 1, the direct inhibition of tendencies ; psychical energy is not called in indirectly by another system of ideas or images ; 2, the production of a large or very large number, according to the circumstances, of accessory physical or psychical phenomena, all in close relationship with the arrest of these tendencies, but imperfectly co-ordinated, and sometimes incoherent ; 3, the entire absorption of the man's psychical energies by the new state of consciousness. This would be still more clearly apparent if we investigated emotions more powerful than those instanced here.

Lastly, a fourth case might be cited ; one in which the emotion produced is extremely strong. If, for example, we unexpectedly lose someone dear to us, or if we receive a very severe injury, a throng of impulses, habits, and psychical systems are suddenly and forcibly arrested in us. The new phenomenon which originates under these extreme conditions presents fresh characteristics : 1, it absorbs all psychical energy ; 2, it culminates in a sort of unconscious condition. The first of these characters is probably the determining condition of the second, for consciousness can scarcely exist when psychical energy is not to some extent distributed.

Thus we find unconsciousness at both ends of the series, although the phenomenon we are studying possesses characteristics that are absolutely opposed. Confining ourselves to the limits within which consciousness and psychical activity are possible, we see that the same characters which we have studied one by one are always encountered. Some of these are always present, whereas any one of the others may be absent from the conditions of an affective phenomenon. These characteristics are the arrest of tendencies, the multiplicity of phenomena, the intensity and persistence of the impulse, the relative lack of co-ordination and the sudden appearance of phenomena, and lastly, the tendency to usurp almost the entire field of consciousness.

As much for the purpose of verifying this law as of

explaining certain phenomena, we should now try to apply it to some groups of well-known facts and show how it may account for them. I shall deal with the matter briefly, since I have already given a considerable number of examples. The abatement and cessation of feeling, for instance, according as an impulse diminishes or ceases, or according as the obstacles disappear, are readily explained. A passage in Tolstoy's *War and Peace* provides a good illustration of the result of this last development, which is not, perhaps, always clearly noted : " It seems to me that you cannot love me ", says Marie to her husband, Nicolas Rostow, " I am so ugly now." " Stop Marie, what nonsense, you ought to be ashamed of yourself. Beauty does not make sweetness, but sweetness makes beauty ; it is only such women as Malvina who are loved for their beauty : do I love my wife ? I don't love her in that way—but ! without you, or even if a black cat should run between us, I feel lost ; I am no longer good for anything. . . . Do I love my finger? . . . Of course not ! I don't love it, but let anyone try to cut it off, that's all ! " In general it would not be said that love no longer exists when that stage is reached. It is, however, certain that love, although it still exists, is very different from what it was originally ; while the greater organization of tendencies and the diminution of impediments are made manifest by this weakening and by a decrease in affective phenomena. Similarly, we find that when the external cause, organic or cerebral, of an impulse is lacking, there is no feeling. Eunuchs have not the same passions as men : a man who leads an inactive, indoor life is less affected by hunger and thirst, other things being equal, than the man who reads, works, or undertakes some physical exercise is when the cessation of other pre-occupations allows these appetites to become apparent. In the same way, we can readily understand why the making of plans is generally accompanied by very perceptible emotions, sometimes keener emotions than those aroused by their realization. The reason is that in the plan the impulse is wholly arrested without being destroyed, while at the same time we find all the circumstances which make for the production of emotion. Further, the emotion is generally strongest at the moment when we are about to achieve our purpose, because then the impulse attains a maximum of strength, whilst for the time being the obstacles still possess the same efficacy.

It is likewise easy to understand why feeling is produced by action associated with that feeling. It is said that Campanella was able to discover what was going on in the mind of a person by imitating his attitude and expression. Hypnotism and artificial sleep are extreme cases of the same thing. "A person whose arms were raised, and who was told that she was being made to bear a burden, imagined that she really had her arms laden with a very heavy weight, and experienced fatigue." "Burke asserts that he often felt the passion of anger kindled within him as he mimicked its external signs, and I do not doubt that in the majority of individuals the same experiment gives the same result."[1] According to Braid,[2] wrinkling the forehead calls up gloomy images, whatever the dominating impression and whatever the organ concerned. The position of the body has a considerable influence upon the emotions and sensations during the period of hypnotic induction ; no matter what passion the hypnotizer is trying to express by means of the patient's attitude, as soon as the necessary muscles are brought into play the passion itself will suddenly burst out, and the entire organization will respond. We cannot fail to recognize in this a good argument for the priority of the tendency of the moment in relation to the production of affective phenomena, and also an

---

[1] Maury, *Le Sommeil et les Rêves*, p. 265. The first instance was taken from Azam and Carpenter, the second from Dugald Stewart.

[2] See Braid, *Neurypnology* (1843) ; also P. Richer, *Études cliniques sur la grande Hystérie*.

unexceptionable instance of the actual effect of the association of movements. An expressive attitude suggests a tendency to a particular system of movements and the system of movements produces the feeling awakened through association by another movement, in the same way and for the same reasons as it produces feeling when it is brought into operation by any other cause.

IV. *Reduction of the various causes to one general cause.—Formula of the general law for affective phenomena*

When we examine and compare all the characteristics which we have recognized as the constant condition of affective phenomena, we can, in my opinion, distinguish a single fact, whose consequences are numerous, as the cause of affective phenomena. The arrest of tendencies, the multiplicity of phenomena, the persistence and strength of impulses, the relative lack of co-ordination, the sudden appearance of phenomena and the tendency to encroach upon the whole field of consciousness—all these are only the effects of a single event, or may even be that event itself ; namely, the liberation of a considerable quantity of psychical energy which cannot expend itself in a systematic manner. Psychical energy is set free in the nerve centres, most frequently under the influence of a stimulus from without : the arrest of the tendency is a sign that this energy cannot expend itself in an harmonious fashion ; there is a want of systematization between the stimulation, the rise of the tendency, and the actual state of the nervous centres and the mind, since the tendency is more or less impeded and prevented from reaching its conclusion. The multiplicity of phenomena, their lack of co-ordination and all the other characteristics are obviously derived from this primary cause, and the affective phenomena in general, emotions, passions, feelings, etc., appear to us, consequently, as the effects of a disturbance of the organism, an ill-co-ordinated state of the physico-psychical phenomena and tendencies; and if we compare affective with intellectual phenomena from the point of view of the peculiar conditions which occasion both, we see that the difference between them lies in the fact that the amount of psychical energy set up is less in the case of the production of the second and the systematization greater. In short, as a complete automatism appears to be the perfect and ideal state of the organism, the intellectual phenomenon is the indication of a slight disturbance and a relatively inconsiderable weakness in systematization, whereas the affective phenomenon is the expression of a more profound disturbance and a more considerable deficiency in systematization and harmony.

This, then, is my definition of the law governing the production of affective phenomena :

An affect is the expression of a more or less profound disturbance of the organism, due to the fact that a relatively considerable quantity of nervous energy is released without being able to be used in a systematic manner. An arrest of the tendencies aroused and a number of physical or psychical phenomena of various kinds, are then produced. At the same time, one or several or all of the following phenomena always appear: persistence of tendencies, relative lack of co-ordination and sudden appearance of the phenomena produced, and the tendency of the awakened impulse to monopolize the field of consciousness.

Chapter II

THE CONDITIONS OF PRODUCTION OF THE DIFFERENT GROUPS OF AFFECTIVE PHENOMENA

I. *Group* i :—*Passions, feelings, affective impulses and signs*

If we examine by means of introspection the data of experience, we discover with a little practice a great many of the elements in our mental life. Some may be perceived without difficulty ; they are clear, strong, exact : such, for example, are, in the intellectual category, our perceptions, and, in the affective, our passions. Others are more obscure, more difficult for entirely untrained minds to observe, and these have been termed weak states of consciousness. Such, for instance, are the images we create of absent objects, and the weak emotions which are revived within us by memory.

Finally, we discover other states, still more vague, with which as a rule thought is very little occupied, except in persons whose nature and occupations lead them to special introspective examination. It is difficult even to give these states an exact name, because they are little known and entirely unclassified : but we may cite as an instance that particular impression which we experience at a time when we are intensely preoccupied with a subject and yet are devoting ourselves to work which is totally unconnected with it and which absorbs nearly the whole of our attention. We no longer think precisely of the object of our preoccupations, nor do we envisage them distinctly, but we are not in the state of mind in which we should be if the preoccupation were

absent. The object of this preoccupation, though absent
from consciousness, is represented there by a peculiar,
unmistakable impression, which often persists for a very
long while in a manner which is appreciable but not clear
to the mind. We may range in this class of phenomena,
also, some of those which Spencer has called relations
between feelings.[1] We ought here to inquire what are
the particular conditions that give rise to the main
groups of affective phenomena, but it is doubtless
advisable to begin with the descriptive part of the subject, and to review those different groups of phenomena
whose conditions we are trying to discover, laying stress
chiefly upon the least known.   It is not my purpose here,
however, to attempt a special descriptive study or to make
a systematic classification of the feelings and passions.

It appears at first sight, perhaps, that we might divide
affective phenomena into groups on the model of a
similar classification of intellectual phenomena, separating them into a number of classes, each of which would
be associated with a corresponding class of cognitive
facts.   But in this way we should obtain only a partially accurate and very imperfect result.   It is true, for
example, that the emotions accompanying those faint
representations which constitute the memory of a person
whose image can arouse emotion within us, are generally
less deep than the emotions which accompany the strong
representations constituting the perception of the same
person.   Nevertheless, that is not always correct ;
there are cases, as we have already seen, which
memory, like imagination, thanks to particular circumstances and to the frame of mind we are in, which allow
only certain sides of the reality to appear, produces an
affective impression stronger than the actual presence.
On the other hand, many cases show that while strong
affective phenomena may accompany weak intellectual
phenomena, very strong intellectual phenomena are
frequently attended by slight emotions or none at all.

[1] v. Herbert Spencer, *Principles of Psychology*, I, p. 163.

Possibly, even, in some cases emotion is produced
without any accompaniment of intellectual phenomena.
We are therefore reduced to working out a general
classification of affects, based solely upon a consideration of the nature of these phenomena and of the
conditions that determine their appearance. Doubtless
an analogous classification of intellectual phenomena
might be made, but the two series would none the
less remain distinct.

The different groups of affective phenomena which I
propose to recognize are : 1, *passions, feelings, affective
impulses* and *affective signs;* 2, *affective sensations;*
3, *emotions.*

The main characteristic of the first group is that it
is produced by tendencies distinguished in some degree
at least by their persistence and their organization.
There is probably no need for me to describe feelings
and passions at length : everybody will understand
sufficiently which are the phenomena that I designate
by these words, to which I attach practically their
ordinary meaning. Then we still have the affective
impulses and affective signs, which it seems to me
necessary to deal with in more detail. Perhaps we
shall explain more clearly the nature of these classes of
facts by referring to intellectual operations. We know
that intellectual phenomena are often substitutes for one
another. Thus the image takes the place of the sensation, the idea or the word may replace the image, the
idea of the word can be a substitute for the word, etc.
This substitution extends farther than is generally
recognized, and the ultimate, most abstract and most
shadowy substitutes have hitherto been seldom studied
by psychologists. I have tried elsewhere to indicate the
part played in language by abstract images, without
colour, tone, sonority, or motive quality, and to define,
to a certain extent, the nature of these images.[1] Such

---

[1] *v.* article by the author : " Le Langage intérieur et la pensée," III,
Revue Philosophique, January, 1886.

representations are pure abstractions, produced, perhaps, by the very weak and systematized partial excitation of a great number of tendencies. We find in the affective sphere facts of substitution analogous to these. Passion and feeling are often replaced by other conscious states of an affective nature, which are substituted for them and play their part. When an image has been often employed and compared with similar images, it vanishes from consciousness, and is replaced by the word, this usually indicating an extension of systematization and a greater facility in intellectual and motor functioning. In the same way, passion and feeling, when for one reason or another they momentarily disappear, may be replaced by a particular substitute which is an affective impulse when the substitute has the effect of directly inducing an action, if it does not encounter too many obstacles, and an affective sign if it results only very indirectly in action and merely forms one element in the formation of other more complex states of consciousness.

For example, it is natural for healthy persons to be hungry at the usual meal-times, when they sit down to table ; but if they are deeply preoccupied, hunger vanishes. Consciousness does not recognize it as hunger properly so-called : and if we mean by the word the phenomenon as it is when the conditions of its appearance are most favourable, hunger is no longer existent. Nevertheless, they eat as much as they would have done under other conditions (assuming that the preoccupation is not too intense), and hunger in this case is replaced by a more or less vague state of consciousness, which is not so definite, perceptible, or strong, but which plays the same part. This is an affective impulse. It is the same with many actions which at the outset have been performed or may sometimes still be performed under the influence of an impulse attended by sufficiently strong feelings. By the force of habit or of particular circumstances they are accomplished without being preceded or attended by this feeling, which is then replaced either by an unconscious tendency or by that somewhat vague affective phenomenon which I call an affective impulse. When we inquire after somebody's health, the question may be accompanied by very different affective phenomena. If it concerns a friend, and we have reasons for disquietude on his account, the inquiry will be accompanied by a rather pronounced affective phenomenon. If the person is of little interest to us, in ordinary circumstances the action will be almost automatic. Lastly, if he be a friend who appears well and hearty, we shall not be very much affected, but neither shall we be entirely indifferent. A phenomenon arises which is not a well-defined feeling — it is not one of uneasiness nor of compassion, nor strictly speaking of tenderness—but nevertheless it may replace one of those feelings and occasion the same words and the same actions. This, again, is an affective impulse.

The affective sign is similar in character. I have already indicated one of the cases in which it is produced. If we have experienced a very strong impression which persists, we may partially dismiss it, but we continually feel within ourselves, not the first impression, but an element temporarily substituted for it, which gives a particular tone to our state of consciousness; we feel that we are quite different from our ordinary selves, without altogether perceiving the cause of the alteration or experiencing any definite feeling, even though the affective phenomenon may be of only a moderate intensity. We must not think, however, that phenomena belonging to the class of substitutes must always be weak. Just as some ideas are stronger than some images, in the sense that they are more conscious, and also in their power to produce actions, so also some affective signs are stronger than some feelings.

We may find other good examples of affective signs in the vague phenomena which are sometimes awakened in association with abstract or very faint images. Lastly, a mental sign which must also be included in this class is the aversion from a person which is left in us by an unpleasant impression formerly experienced and perhaps long-since forgotten, and the vague uneasiness that we feel in his presence. In this last case, the sign remains, but it is no longer understood: its meaning is lost for us.

We have already seen that the general condition of the phenomena belonging to the group we are now studying is that they are due to the arrest of relatively persistent impulses; it must be added that these tendencies have a considerable importance in the psychical or inner life of the individual and in his relations with the outside world—especially the last-named. This is easily explained. A statement of the particular circumstances which accompany the production of each class of phenomena in the first group will connect these phenomena with the general law of the production of affective phenomena and also give us a better understanding of their mutual relations, to which we shall afterwards return.

The passions are the highest manifestation of affectivity; and in order that my metaphors may not be taken literally I would explain that by this I mean that they are affective phenomena in which the characteristics peculiar to affective phenomena in general are stronger than in other phenomena of the same class. In other words, they are those which differ most from non-affective phenomena. We ought, therefore, to find the violent passions exhibiting in an accentuated form all the characteristics that we have successively considered in the preceding parts of this work. In fact, passions are the sign of an extreme disorder in the mutual relations of the different systems that compose the organism and of the organism itself with its environment. We find that they are accompanied to a marked degree by all the phenomena which, as we saw, determine the production of an affective phenomenon. In extreme passion the arrest of tendencies is complete; at the same time, their persistence and intensity are remarkable. I do not think there is any need to dwell upon the phenomena manifested in the appearance of a passion; they can quite easily be analysed and referred to the general laws already indicated. Passion, after all, is generally only the last phase in the evolution of a feeling, and it replaces the feeling when, for one reason or another, the psychical force set in action and not employed in a systematic manner happens to increase. This occurs, for example, when the arrest of tendencies becomes more complete, as when love is intensified by absence. At other times when, the arrest remaining the same, new impulses are added to the first awakened tendencies and operate in the same direction, the shock of the psychical disturbance to the organs and to other mental phenomena increases and sometimes becomes permanent. In these cases one of the most marked characteristics is the invasion of the entire consciousness by the affective phenomenon, and the use of nearly all the available psychical forces in the service of the passion. The extreme results of passion, viz. insanity and death, clearly demonstrate the peculiar violence of the affective phenomenon in its most pronounced manifestations.[1] Here is an example, taken from Letourneau's *Physiologie des passions*, which illustrates extremely well some of the conditions of this mental state; among others, the tendency to invade the entire consciousness, the strength and persistence of the impression, and the disorder and inco-ordination of phenomena. It concerns Alfieri, who says of himself: "I forbade every kind of communication, and I passed the first fortnight uttering dreadful cries and groans. Some friends came to see me; they appeared to pity me. This was, perhaps, because I did not pity myself, but my appearance and demeanour spoke for themselves. I wanted to read, but I could not understand even the newspapers.

[1] *v.* Letourneau, *Physiologie des passions*, Book IV.

Sometimes I would look through whole pages, and read aloud every word, without remembering a single one."[1]

Similarly, when one of the phenomena which conditions passion disappears or decreases in intensity, the passion also disappears and is replaced, according to circumstances, either by a feeling, by indifference, or by a different or opposite passion. The gratification of a passion, that is to say, the diminution of the arrest, generally transmutes it into a feeling. The diminution or disappearance of the tendency brings about the diminution or disappearance of the passion, and sometimes its replacement by an opposite passion. This is shown in violent remorse.

A feeling differs very little from passion except that its phenomena are less intense : the mind is a little more free ; psychical energy is less absorbed ; consciousness is less invaded ; psychical phenomena are weakened and not as a rule very pronounced. Here it is necessary to distinguish feeling from other affective phenomena. The question, in short, is one of classification and nomenclature. Language is very inexact on all these points, largely owing to the readiness with which affective phenomena increase or diminish in intensity, as well as to their frequent complication. Thus, passion and feeling are accompanied, in certain cases, by emotions. In the course of this study I have myself often used the words *emotion* or *feeling* in order to avoid verbal repetition in designating affective phenomena as a whole.[2] But here we must be rigorously exact as to the import of each term, if we wish to establish a classification that shall have any meaning. By feelings (*sentiments*) therefore, I understand those fairly durable

---

[1] Alfieri, quoted by Letourneau, *Op. cit.*, p. 207.

[2] The distinctions here indicated have been preserved as far as possible in translation by rendering *sentiment* as 'a feeling', and taking affective phenomena (*phénomènes affectifs*) as equivalent to 'feeling' in general (=*sensibilité*). *Émotion*, however, always appears as 'emotion', and *passion* as 'passion'. Cf. also footnote to p. 149.—*Trans.*

E

affective phenomena such as ambition, love, fear, hatred, etc., which are less violent than passion and are generally, though not invariably, accompanied by a more or less clear consciousness of their object. There is nothing particular to say about this class of the first group of affective phenomena, except that they possess all the characteristics of passion in a lesser degree ; but these characteristics present themselves less continually and less collectively. Thus, to experience a feeling by no means prevents us from devoting ourselves to a moderately absorbing occupation and from bringing to it sufficient attention to act effectively.

In the affective impulse, the phenomena are still further diminished in intensity. But it is not merely in a general alteration in intensity that the difference consists. When an affective impulse occurs, the tendency arrested is slight, the surplus of psychical energy is inconsiderable, and the concomitant phenomena are very few, but the arrest is almost complete, and the tendency is persistent. This persistence and the strength of the arrest are the only fundamental characteristics of the production of an affective impulse. All the others are very slight. One of them, indeed, is generally absent, namely, the tendency of the affective phenomenon to monopolize consciousness. Here, on the contrary, the field of consciousness is generally occupied by other phenomena, as we saw just now. The affective impulse, in fact, is generally produced when, despite the fact that a great part of the psychical energy is already in operation, a fresh tendency is called up under the influence of some internal or organic excitation, and, though this is checked and cannot manifest itself in action, it nevertheless persists. This is what occurs when we are reading or working, for example, and the desire for movement, exercise, or food, begins to make itself felt, without yet having sufficient strength to make itself an object of attention. Like all the phenomena which we have been examining, the affective impulse is sometimes the product of an arrested tendency, which gives rise to an affective phenomenon of increasing intensity ; and sometimes, on the other hand, the result of the decreasing intensity of the causes that produced a more sharply defined phenomenon of the same order ; or finally, it may be neither preceded nor followed by any other phenomenon of the same order. So, passion may spring from the development of a feeling, or, on the other hand, it may itself give rise to a feeling by a decrease in the intensity of the causes that produce it. Similarly, the affective impulse may be the first step in a psychical process which proceeds from indifference to passion, or, on the other hand, really the outcome of the weakening of a passion or a feeling. We shall have occasion elsewhere to deal at greater length with the subject of the evolution of affects.

The characteristics peculiar to the affective impulse prove that it is more closely akin to a weak intellectual phenomenon or an automatic phenomenon than most affective processes. In fact, intellectual states and states of feeling, which can scarcely be confused in the case of well-defined phenomena (for example, a passion and a reasoning process), bear a singular resemblance to one another when we consider the less differentiated phenomena of each class, just as the animal and the vegetable kingdoms are difficult, if not impossible, to distinguish in the lowest individuals representing them. The intellectual phenomenon and the affective phenomenon actually possess, as we have already had occasion to remark, certain common characteristics, and they are subject to certain common conditions. Now when the differences separating an affective from an intellectual phenomenon are very slight and tend to disappear, as in the case of the affective impulse, or when the phenomena are not very noticeable and are imperfectly differentiated, as in the case of final intellectual substitutes and final affective substitutes, it is obvious that the affective and intellectual phenomena will tend to be confused. Perhaps, indeed, they really are intermingled. Between the abstract idea of hunger and the affective impulse, there is but a slight difference : nevertheless a difference may still be distinguished when the affective character of the impulse is sufficiently pronounced. This difference is probably due to the fact that the impulse is a little stronger when the phenomenon produced is of an affective order, and still more to the fact that in this case it is more persistent. The multiplicity of phenomena is not very evident in the affective impulse : it is, however, frequently displayed in certain physical phenomena—by purposeless movements, such as those in which an awakening impatience is expressed. Inco-ordination of phenomena is, of course, not at all noticeable, neither do they appear abruptly. In all these respects the affective is indistinguishable from the intellectual.

Nevertheless, in my opinion, though the difference is hardly perceptible, in certain circumstances it still exists. It seems to me that I can think of hunger without experiencing an affective impulse ; and, if the circumstances are favourable, the affective impulse is easily aroused.

With the affective sign, the difference in the phenomena becomes even less marked, from the point of view of its end. The affective sign differs from the affective impulse, as we observed, in being unaccompanied by an impulse towards a particular set of movements ; it does not tend directly to produce a movement. As regards its origin, the affective sign, which resembles the affective impulse in all other respects, is distinguished from it, in that the general characteristic of its group— the persistence of the tendency—is weakened, and becomes less constant. The affective sign may be produced by a tendency which persists for a considerable time, or again by a tendency which persists for a relatively short period. Thus it is very difficult to distinguish between the affective sign and the intellectual sign.   In order to become familiar with it we must make use of memory (for direct observation of an affective sign would involve a great risk of the disappearance of the phenomenon and of its replacement by another, an intellectual sign), and compare it with the idea, the abstract mental representation of the same feeling.   We shall see, so far as I can judge—for observation and comparison are not easy—that the two orders of phenomena tend to intermingle, and that even though the affective characteristic, which can hardly be defined or analysed, is still present in one of them only —and this, in my opinion, must be recognized—yet the difference is scarcely perceptible.   With these phenomena we are approaching boundaries within which strict classification is impossible.

Moreover, neither the different classes of affective phenomena, nor even the different classes of psychical phenomena, are separated by well-defined lines, and it is exceedingly difficult to distinguish an intellectual phenomenon from a phenomenon which exhibits the characteristics of affectivity in a very slight degree ; just as it is extremely difficult to distinguish a very powerful feeling from an ordinary passion.   It is generally admitted that every strict classification has a certain artificiality.   There is really not much more in the affective sign than the somewhat brief persistence of a very faint tendency.   The secondary phenomena are greatly weakened : the most persistent, perhaps, are the characteristics of multiplicity and inco-ordination, imperfectly manifested by some physical phenomena. All the other characteristics which accompany the production of a phenomenon of the affective order have vanished, or nearly so ; for, in the most marked cases, the sudden appearance of phenomena may still be found to some extent, but in the least marked cases we come across many faint intellectual indications and instinctive tendencies.

II. *Groups 2 and 3 :—Affective sensations and emotions.*
   General relations of the different classes of affective
   phenomena.

Affective sensations, thus called in order to distinguish
the sensitive from the intellectual element in sensations,
correspond approximately to Spencer's *presentative feel-*
ings, which that author describes as : "mental states
in which, instead of regarding a corporeal impression
as of this or that kind, or as located here or there, we
contemplate it in itself as pleasure or pain : as when
inhaling a perfume."[1]   To this category of affective
phenomena we may also refer all the pleasures of
the senses, considered merely in their sensual aspect.
Affective sensations are distinguished from feelings
in that they are not associated, like the latter, with
very complex groups of tendencies, aiming at the
general systematization of man or of his relations with
his environment.   Thus a feeling such as love, ambition,
or sympathy, or any passion whatsoever, generally has
for cause or for effect the bringing into play of very
complex systems of tendencies and impulses.   This is
never the case with affective sensations ; the tendencies
that awake them are few in number and are less concerned with the deep inner life of the individual, though
they are not unconnected with it, and may have power
to arouse the tendencies which constitute it.

Here, however, affective phenomena of a different
character are produced by the awakening and the
arrest of these new tendencies.   An odour in itself
may seem pleasant to inhale, and if no other psychical
fact happens to be connected with it by association,
it gives us an agreeable sensation.   But if the perfume
reminds us, for instance, of someone we love, and
revives cherished or painful memories, we are very far
from the purely sensual emotion and the affective sensa-

---

[1] Herbert Spencer, *Principles of Psychology*, II, p. 514.

tion. The circle of emotion is widened enormously, and feelings are produced. It is possible to regard the periwinkle as a pretty flower, and to derive a certain mild pleasure from looking at it ; but Rousseau's cry on finding the periwinkle and the emotions called up by the sight of the flower denote affective phenomena very different from the simple affective sensation. From this point of view, even the affective impulse, which is one of the less complex phenomena of the class that we studied first, is still decidedly more complex than the affective sensation. The affective impulse, indeed, is usually the manifestation of a general need of the organism, that is to say of a tendency somewhat complex in its causes, though not necessarily in its effects.

That it is quite otherwise with affective sensations, however, is most clearly shown by the cases in which they (or rather the tendencies which provoke them) produce phenomena of a higher order. I take a striking instance from Guyau : "One summer day, after walking in the Pyrenees until I was completely exhausted, I met a shepherd, and asked him for some milk : he fetched from his cottage, beneath which flowed a brook, a jug of milk which had been standing in water and was of an almost icy temperature. While drinking this new milk, to which the whole mountain had lent its perfume, and which revived me with every delicious draught, I certainly experienced a series of sensations which the word *agreeable* cannot possibly express. It was like a pastoral symphony lingering on the palate, instead of on the ear." [1] Here it is evident that the phenomena have become remarkably complicated : genuine feelings make their appearance—feelings of the contemplative order, in which the tendencies are most speedily arrested ; the least active class, approximating to the affective sensations. We can see how difficult it is to determine the exact limits between groups of phenomena and how little the pure affective

[1] Guyau, *les Problèmes de l'esthétique contemporaine*, p. 63.

sensation differs from the affective sensation accompanied by feeling.

Although a feeling, a passion, an affective impulse, or an emotion may be awakened under the influence of an excitation from without, this excitation only plays a relatively secondary part in the phenomenon. To make use of a familiar comparison, it is the spark which sets fire to the powder; the greater part of the phenomenon is due to the pre-established organization of tendencies. And in the majority of cases the phenomenon may be induced with almost identical characteristics by a different excitation from that which has previously produced it. It is not the same with the affective sensation; here, the excitation from without is relatively of the greatest importance; obviously it could effect nothing without the preliminary organization of the organ which it influences—(it is quite certain that a violet placed in front of a pebble will not produce any affective sensation in the pebble)—but the phenomena to which it gives rise in the organism can only be produced in all their intensity, and with their essential features, by an appropriate excitation.

The phenomena accompanying the production of affective processes exhibit certain peculiarities in the case of an affective sensation. Arrest of tendencies is shown by the fact that habit, by facilitating the relations between the excitation and the organism, diminishes the affective sensation. A pleasant odour ceases to be noticed after a few moments; the pleasure which we feel at the sight of an assemblage of vivid and well-matched colours is somewhat easily dimmed. It is just the same with the pleasure we derive from a combination of sounds which remains unchanged. Perfect harmony is generally agreeable in itself, but, if we listened to it for only five minutes, the pleasure would disappear. An unpleasant affective sensation, then, is often manifested in the place of the pleasant sensation. In this case the phenomenon is doubtless due primarily to local fatigue produced by the excitation ; and if my definition of tendency be recalled, we shall see that here again is another case of a checked tendency. The arrest of the tendency, moreover, is made psychologically evident by the particular circumstance which consists in experiencing a pleasant sensation and delighting in it. When an affective sensation is produced, it is nascent tendencies that are arrested, somewhat as in the case of æsthetic feelings ; indeed, in my opinion, it is impossible to deny the æsthetic character of pleasant affective sensations.

Multiplicity of phenomena in the production of the affective sensation is not very apparent, owing to the fact that the affective phenomenon changes in character and becomes a feeling when too many tendencies and phenomena are evoked. Nevertheless, the affective sensation is attended by a certain diffuse and ill-defined general excitation. This excitation is included in the phenomena which have been described by Féré, in an exceedingly interesting article published in the *Revue philosophique*.[1] Moreover, certain particular phenomena are produced which are determined by the causes we have already recognized. These phenomena are chiefly of the physical kind : imagination is hardly aroused in association with an affective sensation, unless, indeed, the affective sensation is complicated by a feeling. If the affective phenomenon is very pronounced, as in the case of a gourmet eating an artistically prepared dish, the multiplicity of phenomena is accentuated : so, also, is their lack of co-ordination. For instance, there are sighs of satisfaction, exclamations, movements of the head, etc. The most powerful of the affective sensations, sexual enjoyment, is occasionally attended by phenomena which have caused it to be compared with an epileptic fit. The physical phenomena produced are generally directed to the continuance or renewal

[1] Ch. Féré, "Sensation et mouvement", *Revue philosophique*, October, 1885.

of the affective sensation ; such are the movements of the eye or the nostrils, the secretion of saliva, etc., and similar phenomena. We see that here the inco-ordination of phenomena is not at all pronounced. The characteristic of abruptness in appearance is more frequently to be seen. Thus, a colour, or an assemblage of colours, will produce an affective sensation, agreeable or otherwise, which is so much the stronger according as we are the less prepared for it. Even a moderate light causes an unpleasant sensation, if it flashes suddenly upon our eyes as we leave a dark place : and green will appear more beautiful if for some time we have been gazing at red. In short, the tendency of affective phenomena to invade the entire field of consciousness is very evident in the keenest affective sensations. The whole attention can easily be concentrated upon the taste of food, the bouquet of a wine, and the charm of a combination of colours or of sounds (I am here regarding colours and sounds solely as pleasures of the senses—other factors are involved, of course, in music and painting, as we shall have occasion to observe later).

With affective sensations may be associated affective images, which resemble them almost entirely except in vividness and in the fact that they are not caused by an excitation from without. They bear the same relation to affective sensations as intellectual images bear to sensations. They consist in the faint evocation of an affective sensation by memory or imagination. What we may call hallucinations or affective illusions should perhaps be included in this class. For example, when we make a somnambulist drink water by persuading him that he is drinking rum, or cause him to inhale from a bottle which has no scent by telling him that it contains smelling-salts, the phenomena produced may quite well pass for hallucinations or illusions. It may seem strange to use this word in connection with an affective phenomenon. It is true that there can scarcely be a hallucination unless the phenomenon bearing the name is an intellectual one : for error, of which hallucination is an example, is the name we give to a want of systematization in intellectual phenomena. As a matter of fact it is a question of words, but to avoid confusion we must preserve as far as possible the exact significations of our terms and explain why we diverge a little from their ordinary meaning. But, in the matter of the affective sensation and the affective image, intellectual and affective events, though logically distinct, are in reality so closely united that there is scarcely any danger in designating the affective phenomenon by the same name as the intellectual, provided that this is understood beforehand.

Affective images and affective hallucinations comprise a series of phenomena whose intensity increases in proportion to the degree of resemblance they bear to the affective sensation. It is probably unnecessary for me to distinguish affective images from the images that accompany feelings. The distinction would be similar to that which I established between a feeling and an affective sensation. The affective image, like the affective sensation, only concerns the direct data of the senses. It is accompanied, with less intensity, by the same phenomena as the affective sensation. Thus, multiplicity of phenomena shows itself in the first stages of physical phenomena or even in their completed form. The image of the taste of the lemon, for example, at the same time as it produces an affective phenomenon, stimulates the secretion of saliva. I will say nothing more as to the particular characteristics of the affective image in view of their similarity to those we have been studying.

In short, weak substitutes for the affective sensation should still be ranked in the category of affective images, just as we saw in the case of weak substitutes for passion and feeling. I will dwell no further upon this class of phenomena, which is very difficult to observe and which appears to possess no great interest for our further analysis.

We come finally to the third great class of affective phenomena—the emotions: here again we find individual characteristics, which are to be seen in the manifestation of the general causes of affective phenomena. These particular characteristics, as we should expect, are the more evident according as the affective phenomenon itself is more pronounced and differentiated. If we take the case of a powerful and very simple emotion, we shall see these characteristics clearly exhibited.

One of the principal characteristics we observe in emotion is the violence and suddenness of the arrest of tendencies. We experience emotion most keenly when something occurs unexpectedly to disturb the continuity of our mental habits and disorganize our most deep-rooted intellectual tendencies. Thus, if we are curtly informed of the death of someone we love, or receive some other news which tends to sever associations already existing in our mind, we experience an emotion whose violence is proportionate to the suddenness and force of the arrest and the strength and systematization of the arrested tendencies. To love a person means that the image of that person or of his acts—in a word, all that emanates from, and is related, to him—has been attached by innumerable and powerful links to our mental life. The love we feel for a person may be measured by the place which he occupies in our life and by the part played by his words and deeds, or our idea of his sentiments and opinions in the organization of our mental habits—whether this influence be appreciably manifested to consciousness or not. Thus we form systems of ideas, tendencies and impulses which become more and more integrated. The death of the loved one under such conditions is a real disorganization for the one who loves, a rending of self, an arrest of a great number of systems of ideas and tendencies with all the phenomena derived from them. This accounts for the violence of the emotion caused by the news of his death. We can easily see that emotion diminishes according as the arrest is less sudden, and at the same time we can note the difference between emotion and feeling. If, for example, death occurs after a protracted illness, the emotion will be less keen, though the sorrow may be as great and may persist equally long. This is because the knowledge of the illness has already prepared the disorganization of tendencies, and also because new and different tendencies have begun to be formed and have rendered the definitive arrest less sudden.

Everything which in this way augments an impulse or occasions an unexpected arrest, these abrupt nervous discharges which suddenly liberate energy unable to expend itself in a systematic manner, may cause us to experience an emotion. Love which lasts a long time is accompanied by a considerable number of emotions. Whenever anything steps in and discourages or encourages it to a certain extent, that is to say, arrests the growing tendencies or augments them by an initial satisfaction, an emotion is produced. The sight of the loved one, a letter or even some trifling possession, may, in the same way, bring about a sudden liberation of nervous energy which is transferred into an affective phenomenon of the emotional order.

One of the characteristics of emotion, which follows from the above, is its short duration. That an emotion is generally brief is natural enough, since we know that its clearest characteristic is the sudden appearance of phenomena and the emotion is simply the psychical aspect of that appearance. But though emotion is generally of brief duration, it is capable of being renewed ; and, indeed, direct observation seems to show an oscillation between emotion and non-emotion, whenever the first emotion has been very sharp. From an almost uniform background of sorrow or joy, which indicates the persistence of the tendency

or of the arrest, emotive phenomena are abruptly
detached from time to time, sometimes under the influence of an accessory idea which happens to be
awakened, sometimes without any appreciable cause.
Grief or joy is intensified from time to time, suddenly
and for a comparatively short period, and then
diminishes. It is unnecessary to add that the sudden
appearance of the arrest, and the brevity of the emotion,
may on some occasions be more marked than others.

Emotion is often produced by an external stimulus:
a letter we are reading, an encounter, a shock, or a
sudden impression, visual or auditory. But we have
already seen that in this respect an emotion is distinguished from an affective sensation in that it is
certainly less directly linked to the cause which gives
rise to it, and that the organico-psychical conditions
of the development of emotion are much more complex
and profound than in the case of affective sensation.
Moreover, an idea, as well as a sensation, may give
rise to a very strong emotion. For this to happen
the idea has only to occur unexpectedly and to be
accompanied by the awakening of a tendency which is
sharply arrested or which shows a powerful tendency
to arrest others.

Multiplicity of phenomena is a very pronounced feature in emotions, and emotion is particularly exhibited
through exceedingly numerous physical phenomena;
among these, as we have seen, are increased or de-
creased secretions, or modifications of their nature.
According to Maudsley, there is not a single nutritive
act that emotion cannot affect. The physical effects of
fear, surprise, unexpected disgrace, and the like, are
very clear and well known. The action exerted upon
the heart is very important, and may even occasion
death. In short, strong emotion exhibits, in a remarkably intense form, all the characteristics which we
enumerated above when dealing with the general causes
of affective phenomena.

Multiplicity is much less noticeable in association with psychical phenomena. So long as emotion lasts, it produces a sort of psychical inhibition : the mind is as though paralyzed and becomes incapable of imagination, reasoning, and even sensibility, except in so far as the emotion itself is concerned.

Consequently, we find here in a high degree the tendency to invade the entire field of consciousness, which we have indicated as a characteristic of a great number of affective phenomena. The present case has one peculiarity : consciousness is not invaded by a system of psychical facts, but by a single impression.

Multiplicity of phenomena and the tendency to invade the entire field of consciousness are not contradictory, as one might at first suppose. In fact, at the outset, the tendency to occupy consciousness may be manifested without the disappearance of all the other conscious phenomena, and of course it is quite compatible with the appearance of a great number of physical phenomena. In short, as we have seen, if the tendency to absorb all the psychical forces reaches its highest degree, if the whole field of consciousness is invaded by a single impression, consciousness ceases, and emotion, so far as it is a state of consciousness, disappears also. That is to say, as a rule, although the tendency to encroach upon the field of consciousness makes itself felt to a certain extent, it does not completely attain its end.

During emotion, which is a kind of mental shock even when it is relatively weak, consciousness is almost entirely engrossed—occasionally to the extent of becoming less clear, the mind undergoing a kind of transient obfuscation. "A veil passed before my eyes", is a formula frequently used to depict this state of mind. I could cite numerous passages from various works of fiction in which the same phenomenon is described. "To be stupefied", "to lose knowledge of things", "to be dazzled", are expressions that are very appositely employed for the description of a sufficiently strong emotion.

These characteristics are perfectly indicated in the description of emotion given by Letourneau. Although Letourneau appears to use the word emotion in a less precise sense than that which I myself adopt, the characteristics which he enumerates and presents here can scarcely belong to anything but emotion, as I understand it.

"The brain, reeling from the effects of a severe moral blow, is alive to nothing else. Nervous activity is concentrated upon one point, and consequently there is a more or less complete interruption of the relations between the nervous centres and the other organs. The voluntary muscles, forgotten by the cerebro-spinal axis, are debilitated—sometimes made powerless. The legs give way; an athlete for the time being is weaker than a child. The organs of the special senses become practically useless : the ear no longer hears, the eyes no longer see. It is then possible to be severely hurt or mutilated and yet to feel scarcely anything.

"The organic functions do not escape the general disorder. The heart, which has a double nerve supply (parasympathetic and sympathetic) and whose muscle fibres are striated, is first upset. Sometimes the heartbeats are quickened for a moment, but soon they slacken, and often stop ; hence the accompanying pallor and occasionally the fainting fit. Respiration, of course, shares the fate of the circulation. The secretions are disturbed ; the work of digestion is checked. Like the other muscles, the paralyzed sphincters are relaxed: they even lose their tone.

"Intellectual functions are, of course, almost suspended, whether there is faintness or not. It is impossible to apply oneself to anything that is extraneous to the impression of the moment. But this period of depression is of short duration. The tide of life, momentarily checked or abated, rushes on apace and an energetic reaction is produced.

" The concentration of nervous activity is followed by a great expansion. The muscular system again becomes active, and may even acquire astonishing power. The senses awaken, but the attention still holds fast to a single idea and will not allow the exhausted individual to perceive anything that has not some bearing upon the emotion. The intellectual faculties, likewise, can function energetically only in the direction of the moral impression. For the same reason, there is still partial or entire insensibility to physical pain.

" The pulsations of the heart, feeble at first, become violent, rapid and tumultuous. The brain is congested, the face swollen and flushed, the respiration hurried, panting. Secretions are formed with abnormal activity. Tears often flow in abundance : frequently a flood of bile is poured into the intestines. The whole of the gastro-intestinal glandular apparatus is probably affected ; for there is often vomiting, etc. In the nursing mother, the lacteal secretion, which is generally suspended by emotion, is not invariably re-established.

" Sometimes the kidneys secrete an enormous quantity of colourless, watery urine. If bile is secreted in too great a quantity to be speedily expelled, it is re-absorbed and there is jaundice. Sweat is generally abundant.

" . . . At the end of a usually fairly short period, the inordinate organic excitation caused by the emotion dies away, leaving in its train the weariness and depression which always follow excessive expenditure of energy."

The emotions form a class of affective phenomena which has the noteworthy characteristic of accompanying other affective phenomena. They correspond to an abrupt change in the mode of action and strength in the power of the tendencies whose arrest produces a feeling or a passion. Love, hatred, ambition and the like are accompanied by emotions, as we have seen,

F

when some occurrence favours or hinders them. Emotions, therefore, possess a rational character more obvious than that of other phenomena of the same kind. In the same class as emotions, we must include pleasure and pain, which nevertheless ought to be considered separately. They share with the emotions the characteristic of being, to a higher degree than other affective phenomena, concomitant or accompanying states, and they hardly exist independently of the states of feeling or intelligence which accompany them. There are different tones, which nearly all feelings, passions, and emotions, are capable of assuming, according to the degree of systematization of the tendencies that produce them. Pleasure is the result of a growing systematization ; pain is the result of a decreasing systematization : both of course imply, as do all affective phenomena and indeed all conscious events, that the systematization is imperfect. It is also apparent that the concomitants of such a feeling as love or hate vary in relation to the pleasure or pain of the moment, the nature and strength of the check sustained by the tendencies which produce it, and the degree of harmony between these tendencies and the previous habits of the brain and the general disposition.

Nevertheless, in one way pleasure and pain differ remarkably from other emotions : they are capable of lasting much longer, and the sudden appearance of phenomena is not more pronounced in their case than in the generality of affective phenomena. As they may accompany practically all other affective phenomena, it follows that they possess scarcely any peculiar characteristic other than the above.

Lastly, by way of concluding this chapter, we may observe incidentally that emotion, like other affective phenomena, can be more or less intense, and that its weaker and more slightly differentiated forms may easily be confused with the weaker forms of the phenomena we examined earlier. In every case, after the insensible degradation of the characteristics that give an affective phenomenon its individuality, we obtain a sort of psychological residue, which is not a bare abstraction, since consciousness can recognize it, but which it is unnecessary to study at greater length, since it seems to have no particular properties except the weakening of the causes that give rise to the phenomenon and the correlative weakening of the phenomenon produced.

SUMMARY OF THE TWO FIRST CHAPTERS

PRINCIPAL GROUPS

AFFECTIVE PHENOMENA in general

General conditions

Liberation of psychical energy which cannot be employed in a systematic way and expressed by sufficiently co-ordinated phenomena.

———

Essential Phenomena

Arrest of tendencies.

Multiplicity of phenomena.

———

Secondary Phenomena

Not always appearing all at once, but one at least being necessary in the production of the affect.

Relative inco-ordination of phenomena.

Sudden appearance of phenomena.

Persistence of the impulse.

Intensity of the impulse.

Tendency to monopolize the field of consciousness almost entirely, and to absorb nearly the whole of the psychical forces.

DIVISIONS

GROUP I

General characters

1. Persistence of impulses.

2. Complexity and considerable importance of the tendencies brought into play.

SUBDIVISIONS

1. Passions

Extreme intensity of the impulse.

Very strong tendency to invade consciousness and to absorb the psychical forces. Pronounced inco-ordination in extreme cases.

2. Feelings

The same characteristics in a lower degree.

3. Affective Impulses

and

4. Affective Signs

Inco-ordination of phenomena very slightly marked. Tendency to absorb the psychical forces very weak. Decrease, especially in connection with affective signs, of the persistence of impulses. Approach of weak phenomena of a purely intellectual order and of weak phenomena appertaining to other classes of affective phenomena.

GROUP II.—Affective Sensations

General characters

1. Specialized excitation from without, playing a preponderant part in their appearance.

2. Rapid weakening and weak persistence of the tendency which calls up the affect.

3. Slight complexity and organic importance of the tendencies brought into play.

4. Multiplicity of phenomena, for the most part comparatively slightly marked. The weak forms progressively approach the weak forms of the other groups.

GROUP III.—Emotions

General characters

1. Sudden liberation of nervous energy and sudden appearance of phenomena.

2. Very slight duration of the mode of psychical activity which produces the emotion.

3. Multiplicity of phenomena manifested especially by physical phenomena.

4. Complete absorption of psychical forces.

Character highly rational. Manifested above all in concomitance with other affective phenomena.

Pleasure and pain are connected with this group by the relational character they possess in a high degree, without preserving the other characteristics of the group.

There are slight varieties of emotion, characterized by the weakening of the characters indicated. The weakest forms approximate to weak kinds of other groups of affective phenomena or even psychical phenomena, or are confused with them.

CHAPTER III

THE LAWS OF PRODUCTION OF
COMPOUND AFFECTIVE PHENOMENA

I. *The position of the problem*

WE have dealt so far with the circumstances determining
the production of affective phenomena in general or of
a particular group, without concerning ourselves with
the simplicity or complexity of the phenomenon produced. We have merely observed that the multiplicity
of phenomena and the awakening of a number of
tendencies are permanent characteristics of the appearance of an affect without insisting upon the fact that
the rise of new tendencies produces new affective
phenomena, when those tendencies are to some extent
checked in their development, as is frequently the case.
Similarly, we have ignored the fact that often, perhaps
under the influence of two distinct causes, two opposite
or at least entirely different impulses occur, and that the
different affective phenomena which result combine to
give a special character to the synthetic state of consciousness which is then produced. Such are the
compound affective phenomena which are occasioned,
for example, by the performance of an opera, or, more
simply, by listening to an air with an accompaniment
which has a different character from that of the song :
as, for example, the serenade in Don Juan. This kind
of effect is produced by a method frequently employed
in dramatic music, which consists in the repetition by
the orchestra of a *motif* previously heard in a different
situation, associating it with other impressions than
those which we would naturally feel while listening to

it. Lastly, an affective phenomenon is produced by an
arrested tendency, but this tendency is generally checked
by the action of other tendencies which also sustain
arrest, and, if this arrest is sufficiently powerful, it is
easy to understand that opposite feelings arise simultaneously in the mind. If, for example, the idea of theft
occurs to an honest man who is destitute, the nascent
tendency is checked by the mental habits he has
acquired : but these habits are more or less forcibly
impaired by the incipient idea. Reference to the definition of tendency which I gave at the beginning of the
first chapter will show that this also is an arrest of
tendency. Hence a complex state of consciousness
arises, a result of shame, of longing, of dignity, of
apprehension ; of hunger, perhaps ; of misery, etc. All
these will be more or less amalgamated into a single
state of consciousness, and the various feelings resulting
from the various tendencies may alternately occupy the
'visual point' of consciousness. But even in this case,
the conditions which are momentarily effaced do not
entirely disappear. The total state of consciousness
derives from them a particular tone ; and at other times,
indeed, it seems that two feelings unite without mingling
and that, as in the 'luxury of pity' and the 'luxury of
grief', which we shall have occasion to consider more
closely, the feeling is in some measure twofold.

A complex affect may present itself, consequently,
under different forms and with greater or less unity.
There are cases in which the various tendencies are
so completely harmonized that consciousness seems to
be occupied by a single feeling and it is necessary to
study it attentively and decompose it by analysis or
re-combine and vary it by synthesis, in order to realize
its complexity. In other cases, on the contrary, it seems
that the mind experiences two feelings at the same time.
The contrast between the phenomena is just sufficiently
plain to be perceived clearly by consciousness. At
other times consciousness is in a state of extreme

agitation, resulting from the struggle between two tendencies of almost equal power which cannot co-exist and are both trying to attract the psychical forces to themselves. Lastly, certain persons at any rate possess tendencies which are so strong, well-organized and bound up with all or nearly all the systems of tendencies which make up the organism, that no opposing tendency can wage serious warfare upon them, or attract to itself enough psychical energy to become manifest in consciousness. We must study in succession these various general complex forms of affective phenomena, and try to determine their laws.

II. *The non-unified forms of complex affective phenomena*

It is a well-known fact that an individual includes within himself a certain number of tendencies, of systematized associations which, though opposed to each other, may co-exist and manifest themselves either successively or simultaneously. Man possesses neither metaphysical unity (the meaning of which, in any case, is very vague), nor even physiological functional unity.[1] A most curious phenomenon which offers a good example of man's lack of unity, is a fact established by psychological experimentation, which illustrates the completely independent operation of several systems of motor tendencies. Speaking of a subject in a state of somnambulism, Richer observes: "the patient may be shared by two experimenters, between whom connection is maintained only through the half of the body which each is working upon. The sphere of action of the two experimenters is perfectly delimited by a vertical sagittal plane passing through the middle of the body of the subject. Each of them can move his hands over one half of the body—face, back, chest, even under the garments, without provoking

[1] See article by the author upon the variations of personality in the normal state, *Revue philosophique*, May, 1882.

any gesture or prohibitory motion; but directly the operator's hand crosses the median line, B. moans and recoils in order to avoid the touch of the hand which exceeds the limits of the territory allotted to it.

" Each of the experimenters can at will produce contractions by a puff of breath or by passes, but only in the half of the body he is controlling. In the same way, a contraction caused by one experimenter cannot be counteracted by the other; for example, the experimenter on the left cannot exert any influence over a contraction produced on the right by the other experimenter.

"Pressure upon the vertex, exerted by a fresh experimenter, changes the state of affairs immediately and gives the new-comer all power of producing the various phenomena of somnambulism." [1]

Taine has given an account of a very curious and well-known fact, in which we again find a creation of a distinct dual personality. The subject writes, without being aware of it.

"I have seen a person who, while talking and singing, writes coherent sentences and even whole pages without looking at her paper or being conscious of what she is writing. In my opinion she is completely sincere; and she declares that at the end of the page, she has no idea of what she has written; when she reads it, she is astonished, sometimes alarmed. The handwriting is different from her ordinary script. The movements of her hands and of the pencil seem automatic. The writing always ends with the signature of some dead person, and it is in the nature of intimate thoughts rising from hidden mental deeps which the author would not willingly divulge. This is certainly a case of dual personality, of the simultaneous presence of two parallel and independent series of ideas, of two centres of action, or, if you will, two personalities simultaneously occupying in the same brain, each at its

[1] Richer, *Études cliniques sur l'hystéro-épilepsie.*

work and each at different work, one on the stage, the other in the green-room : the second as complete as the first, since, alone and unnoticed it forms coherent ideas and writes down connected phrases, in which the first has no share."[1]

It is legitimate to ask, with reference to this last observation, whether the subject may be said to have no consciousness of that deep mental recess, or whether it is not, as Taine suggests, rather a question of an entire dissociation of psychical systems. In that case, each system would form a kind of ego, and, though quite conscious in itself, would not be apparent to the consciousness of the other. One of these systems would be for a while in direct dynamic communication with the organs that govern handwriting ; the other would be connected with the speech-organs. It is certainly difficult to prove directly the reality of the psychical phenomena accompanying the nervous process which terminates in the act of writing, but the actual fact of writing may be considered as supplying at least a strong presumption in favour of the theory which admits dual consciousness in the literal sense. It must be remembered that proof of the existence of a conscious event is never direct, for only by induction can we believe in the existence of consciousness in others. One thing, I believe, will then be apparent : whatever the difference between the reasons leading to the induction that facts of consciousness in the preceding case accompany the physiological process ending in speech, and those which incline us to allow that facts of consciousness also accompany the physiological process which has its outcome in writing, that difference is nevertheless not great enough to permit our rejecting

[1] *De l'Intelligence*, 4th edit., Preface, p. 16. See also some curious experiments of Dumontpallier, in the contribution entitled "Indépendance fonctionnelle de chaque hémisphère cérébral " (illusions and unilateral hallucinations provoked in the hysterical) *Comptes rendus des séances et mémoires de la Société de biologie*, 1882, p. 786. For a complete account of the question, see Ribot, *Les Maladies de la personnalité*.

this latter hypothesis altogether. Moreover, the solution of the question does not vitally concern us.

In normal life we frequently come across analogous facts, though they are not so striking; the systems of dynamic associations which simultaneously come into play are less dissociated, but in certain cases we find almost a reflection of the pathological phenomenon. This occurs, for example, when we write while thinking of something else or while talking to a friend. A kind of reduplication of the self takes place, which may be quite pronounced. A similar phenomenon emerges in the case of the pianist who has to make different movements with his two hands according to the signs for the notes which have a different meaning in the treble and bass clefs. Obviously, in this case the attention can be divided to a certain extent, but we cannot doubt that in the process of division it is lessened. To be able to play a difficult piece at sight requires long practice; and when we talk while we are writing, we run the risk of making mistakes either in what we are saying or what we are writing or in both. Nevertheless consciousness may undoubtedly persist, though somewhat obscured, and be applied to two actions at the same time.

In relation to affective phenomena, the problem may be stated thus: can the mind experience two different feelings at the same time, and can it synthesize them in one state of consciousness?

The first question concerns us less than the second. Indeed, if we experienced two isolated and unrelated feelings we should have no reason for regarding them as a compound feeling, and the study of such phenomena, curious as they may be in themselves, does not fall within the compass of our present investigation. But it would be interesting, in order to embrace the whole series of phenomena whose extreme limits do not directly concern us, to take first the affective phenomena which are entirely distinct, then those which are readily associated and adapted to one another, at first badly, then better,

then well, and, finally, to take those which are completely harmonized and which, like the other end of the
series, also fall outside the scope of study. It would be
useless, however, to dwell at length upon the occurrence
of separate affective phenomena existing in the same
organism for two distinct consciousnesses. Nothing
certain, or even probable, can be said at present.

We have already seen that several circumstances may
bring about the simultaneous production of different
affective phenomena. Let us take these circumstances
one by one and see what happens when they are present.
There is a certain unity in every conscious event. This
unity, whose cause we need not inquire into (the dynamic
association of nervous elements), is very obvious, and
easily masks the diversity of the phenomena making up
the state of consciousness. If we examine it carefully, however, we can, by introspection alone, eventually
discover the elements which are united into a more or
less co-ordinated whole. Thus, some persons make a
very complex impression upon us ; we feel a certain
liking for them, and some of their qualities even inspire
in us a certain respect, while at the same time we are
repelled by other aspects of their personality. According as the balance inclines to the side of sympathy or
antipathy or apparently to neither, we say that the
person makes a pleasing, displeasing, or indifferent
impression upon us. But these statements are crude
and only approximate. In reality, it nearly always, if
not always, happens that in one and the same person
certain qualities please us, others displease us ; others,
maybe, please and displease us at the same time ; and,
lastly, some leave us completely indifferent. But since
we have to consider as a single whole the combination
of qualities which are never separated from one another,
at any rate in actuality, it follows that our impression,
when we think of the person, is complex and sometimes
very indefinite. Usually we find that according to
our particular state of mind at the moment, the inclina-

tion to sympathy or to antipathy gets the better of us, but the feelings we neglect are never wholly absent from consciousness or, at any rate, very rarely, and in certain instances they quite perceptibly co-exist. We therefore feel at the same time attracted and repelled. The total state of consciousness is an imperfect synthesis of contrary elements; sympathy and antipathy are to some extent co-existent. The general impression loses its definiteness, it is less clear than when the elements of the state of consciousness are in perfect agreement, and, so far as I can see, a certain mental constraint is always experienced: this comprises a new affective element which is added to the others.

Furthermore, we may cite the case in which a sad occurrence causes mirth, or a happy event sorrow. This is not rare, and it is a recognized fact that there is no such thing as unmixed joy. Yet it would be a mistake to think that an average is struck between joy and sorrow, and that, for example, when a sad event is accompanied by some circumstances which please us, the pleasure diminishes our original grief and that our sorrow is diminished by the amount of pleasure the new circumstances have occasioned. I do not say that an effect of this kind is never produced, but it is not always produced; and never, moreover, do matters proceed with such mathematical exactitude. The "smile that shines through tears" corresponds to a complex state of feeling: it plainly signifies that the mind, for the time being, experiences a complex emotion composed of sad and pleasant elements; and no one surely would maintain that at the precise moment when an unhappy person smiles at a little child, the feeling of sadness completely vanishes from consciousness, leaving the entire domain free for a cheerful feeling, which in its turn will suddenly disappear and permit fresh manifestation of grief.

In short, certain complex conditions of this description are so frequent that their elements have come to adapt themselves to one another and co-exist undisturbed in consciousness.   Such is melancholy, which has been defined as "the happiness of being sad " : such, again, are the feelings which Spencer refers to as the 'luxury of pity' and the 'luxury of grief'.

In nearly all the examples we have just cited, to which we shall have to return in order to explain and analyse them, we find this common characteristic : the feeling always has a well-defined quality of unity ; by that I mean that the affective phenomena, varied as they may be, are related to the same subject, that is to say, to a single powerfully-organized group of perceptions, images and intellectual signs.

It may be otherwise, and in connection with affective impulses we have seen a case in which the phenomenon is produced under somewhat different conditions.   In this case, consciousness is partially occupied by an affective phenomenon which bears no relation to the object which is pre-eminently occupying it at the moment.   This condition arises, for example, when our attention is a little distracted from some occupation by the need for food, or when the mind admits, without appreciable cause, a pleasant recollection in a moment of sorrow or a gloomy idea in a moment of joy, though the causes of the pleasant and the painful emotions may have no other apparent connection than simultaneity.   Here again, in some cases, there is a combination of feelings ; but this does not always happen.   That such a combination is possible is proved by the fact that we can experience the truth of Dante's lines : *Nessun maggior dolore* . . .

"No greater grief than to remember days
    Of joy, when misery is at hand . . ."[1]

If Musset contradicted this with arguments which sometimes approached the fantastic, and without always appearing to understand it aright, the explanation is

[1] *Inferno*, V, 121-123.

that he was not experiencing the phenomenon when he wrote his *Souvenir*. Indeed, it does not by any means always occur, but it is none the less real in those who experience it, and actually many do.

At other times, on the contrary, the two phenomena remain apart. Thus the affective impulse of hunger, which may co-exist in the mind with acute grief, with a feeling of love, ambition, etc., is not at all liable to be confused with that feeling. The two phenomena are very clearly recognized by consciousness as being different and simultaneous, and the evidence of this is that sometimes a conflict is set up in the mind between the two, a struggle of which we are fully conscious. Frequently, indeed, the contest between the two feelings causes the awakening of a third affective phenomenon, regret, shame, etc.

The phenomena which arise in the case of a more or less complete and clear distribution of consciousness and attention among several affective facts are therefore numerous and varied. An analysis of the causes should enable us to explain them and refer them to their laws.

We will examine successively the three principal cases which have already been enumerated. In the first place, two different excitations of the organs of vegetative life, coming from outside or arising in the brain without apparent cause, may bring into play tendencies belonging to different systems of psychical associations, which are almost wholly unconnected. To return to an example already cited : if we experience the first pangs of hunger or thirst while we are reading or travelling, the different impulses that these tendencies arouse are scarcely capable of combining in any degree. Each seeks to draw to it itself the psychical forces, according to a law which we have recognized ; but before either prevails, both are actually present in consciousness, for a longer or shorter time. A somewhat complex state then arises, comprising the two tendencies, plus a feeling of relationship between the two which often imparts an affective tinge — regret, tedium, anxiety, etc. In this case the two tendencies do not appear to blend in a single distinct phenomenon. Consciousness, if it is exerted at all, quite easily recognizes at the same time two distinct affective phenomena ; and the impossibility of synthesizing them into a harmonious system causes the partly unpleasant general impression resulting from the struggle between the two systems, and further complicates the original state of affairs. In the production of this third emotion, we may observe, by the way, the arrest of tendencies and lack of systematization which always accompany the production of affective phenomena, whatever the degree of complexity possessed by the factors. Here once more the emotion is due, as always, to a failure to effect systematization.

But it would be a mistake to suppose that the concomitant phenomena and opposite tendencies cannot be manifested at the same time without entering into conflict and giving rise to additional emotions. In fact, though we admit that there is in every organism a tendency to systematization—and experience compels us to recognize this—this tendency is not always manifested with the same intensity and in the same manner. I mean that phenomena are not always—it might even be said that they are never—wholly co-ordinated and unified with regard to their ends. So we see diametrically opposed characteristics persisting in the same individual. I know, of course, that it is sometimes a superior form of organization which allows this or that tendency, according to circumstances, to be produced for the good of the individual ; but it is also very often a flaw in organization, for we cannot always say that this lack of harmony in the individual corresponds to a lack of harmony in the conditions of existence. It may have been engendered by the latter, but very often it is for the organism a cause, not of more complete and varied adaptation, but of confusion and decadence.

To come back to our case: there is certainly a lack of harmony when we are swayed between the desire to continue a piece of work and the necessity for restoring our energy ; but this lack of harmony may be weakened as far as consciousness is concerned. We can accustom ourselves to work with pleasure, while perceiving in the dim portion of our consciousness affective tendencies or affective signs that tend to divert us from our occupation. That may result from two different causes: either the main occupation is so absorbing and uses up so much psychical energy that the affective phenomenon derived from an opposite tendency remains weak, too weak to struggle with the first tendency, or else habit has imposed on the mind the simultaneous presence of two phenomena which differ in intensity, and neither tendency appears to absorb the strength of the other: the two systems remain almost entirely separate, and the only relations between them are those which will enable them to be present in consciousness at the same time. Thus, *the separation of tendencies and the absence of conflict between them are the conditions under which two affective phenomena may be present in consciousness, without a third affective phenomenon being produced. On the contrary, tendencies belonging to separate but conflicting systems produce a new affective phenomenon in accordance with the general laws we have formulated; and this new phenomenon is added to the others and makes the state of consciousness still more complex.*

The facts we have quoted illustrate the working of the law which we have just stated. We will give an example, to recall the different forms of the phenomenon successively produced by the same process.

In a burning room a man is working to save from the flames the things he values most highly: so long as he can breathe freely, the organic tendency manifested in breathing and the psycho-organic tendency manifested in feelings of anguish, fear, haste, etc., occur at the same time; and one of them only is represented by phenomena of the conscious and affective order. When breathing begins to be difficult, it forces itself into consciousness. Nevertheless, the two tendencies persist without yet entering into conflict: the systems of phenomena, which hitherto were without perceptible dynamic association, begin, thanks to the irradiation of nervous effects (inhibition, dynamogenesis, various reflexes), to combine to a sufficient extent to participate at the same time in the same state of consciousness. At length, when the discomfort grows more and more pronounced, and the irradiation and diffusion of nervous effects become greater and greater, each system makes too heavy a claim upon the psychic forces. The strife among the tendencies extends to the feelings which accompany them, and the state of consciousness grows more and more complicated, until one of the tendencies, that one of the dynamic combinations which is least organized, is conquered, and for the time being no longer manifests itself with sufficient intensity to give rise to affective phenomena.

The second mode of appearance of compound affective phenomena less frequently produces ill-systematized and almost unrelated phenomena. Nevertheless, it produces fairly easily affects of absolutely opposite characters, pleasure and grief, for example, and even feelings which seem to be contradictory, such as approval and displeasure. The phenomena in this class manifest a higher degree of harmony and less conflict between opposite elements than any other composite affective phenomena. Sometimes, indeed, as we shall have occasion to observe, conflict becomes an element of harmony.

The same event or the same person may arouse in the mind opposite tendencies which are generally related to one another, since they are part of the same psychical system; and opposite tendencies may be accompanied by affective phenomena which will naturally present

G

contrary characteristics. In other cases an arrested tendency may awaken by association other diversified tendencies, whose activity will again create two different groups of phenomena. Here, therefore, we have two sets of circumstances, in which the same excitation evokes two different tendencies and indirectly creates two opposite affective phenomena which become more or less blended.

Here again, however, we find cases in which the different feelings are to a greater or lesser extent amalgamated. Sometimes the compound state of consciousness attains to a high degree of cohesion and unity, although it may be composed of opposite elements. Furthermore, it is sometimes one of these opposite elements which engenders the other : a pleasure gives rise to a pain, a pain to a pleasure, and the two are so unified within our consciousness that they can scarcely be decomposed. At other times, opposition may inspire respect, and so on. In cases where the compound phenomenon does not admit elements so intimately united, the two affects are not engendered by one another, but are produced separately in consciousness, and are united by a less perfect synthesis. We will begin as before with the case in which the harmony and synthesis of affective phenomena of opposite character come nearest to perfection.

It is to this class that we must assign the luxury of pity and the luxury of grief which we mentioned before and which we will now examine in detail.

"There is", says Spencer, "a pleasurably-painful sentiment, of which it is difficult to identify the nature, and still more difficult to trace the genesis. I refer to what is sometimes called ' the luxury of grief '.

" It seems possible that this sentiment, which makes a sufferer wish to be alone with his grief, and makes him resist all distraction from it, may arise from dwelling on the contrast between his own worth as he estimates it and the treatment he has received—either from his fellow-beings or from a power which he is prone to think of anthropomorphically. If he feels that he has deserved much while he has received little, and still more if instead of good there has come evil, the consciousness of this evil is qualified by the consciousness of worth, made pleasurably dominant by the contrast. One who contemplates his affliction as undeserved, necessarily contemplates his own merit as either going unrewarded, or as bringing punishment instead of reward : there is an idea of much withheld, and a feeling of implied superiority to those who withhold it.

" If this is so, the sentiment ought not to exist where the evil suffered is one recognized by the sufferer as nothing more than is deserved. Probably few, if any, ever do recognize this ; and from those few we are unlikely to get the desired information. That this explanation is the true one, I feel by no means clear. I throw it out simply as a suggestion : confessing that this peculiar emotion is one which neither analysis nor synthesis enables me clearly to understand."[1]

Spencer's explanation appears to me ingenious, and I believe that it may account for certain particular cases ; but it is not sufficiently general to explain every case of the 'luxury of grief'. This pleasure caused by the existence of grief may also be manifest when suffering appears to be a just reward of conduct. There is a certain pleasure in submitting voluntarily to a punishment known to be deserved ; and it is not without pleasure, perhaps, that very pious people meet certain afflictions which they deem to be sent by God and which they cannot condemn as unjust. I am now going to suggest a general explanation of these facts, including the 'luxury of pity', in connection with which I shall again quote Spencer's description and his explanation which, like the other, is ingenious but incomplete. "Under its primary form, pity implies simply the representation of a pain, sensational or

[1] Spencer, *Principles of Psychology*, Vol. II, pp. 590-591.

emotional, experienced by another ; and its function as so constituted, appears to be merely that of preventing the infliction of pain, or prompting efforts to assuage pain when it has been inflicted. In this process there is implied nothing approaching to pleasure—relief from pain is all the pitying person gains by gaining it for the person pitied. But in a certain phase of pity the pain has a pleasurable accompaniment ; and the pleasurable pain, or painful pleasure, continues even where nothing is done, or can be done, towards mitigating the suffering. The contemplation of the suffering exercises a kind of fascination—continues when away from the sufferer, and sometimes so occupies the imagination as to exclude other thoughts. There arises a seemingly abnormal desire to dwell on that which is intrinsically painful—a desire strong enough to cause resistance to any distraction : a resistance like that which the luxury of grief causes. How does there originate this pleasurable element in the feeling? Why is there not in this case, as in other cases, a readiness, and even an eagerness, to exclude a painful emotion? Clearly we have here some mode of consciousness which the foregoing explanations overlook."[1]

The problem is well stated. We would merely observe that Spencer seems to allow too readily a complete finality to the organization of the mind and to be unduly surprised at finding facts which contradict this idea. Here is his solution :

"All those cases where the luxury of pity is experienced, are cases where the person pitied has been brought by illness or by misfortune of some kind to a state which excites this love of the helpless. Hence the painful consciousness which sympathy produces, is combined with the pleasurable consciousness constituted by the tender emotion. Verification of this view is afforded by sundry interpretations it yields. Though the saying that 'pity is akin to love' is not

---

[1] Spencer, *op. cit.*, Vol. II, pp. 622-623.

true literally, since in their intrinsic natures the two are quite unlike, yet that the two are so associated that pity tends to excite love, is a truth forming part of the general truth above set forth. That pleasure is found in reading a melancholy story or witnessing a tragic drama, is also a fact which ceases to appear strange. And we get a key to the seeming anomaly, that very often one who confers benefits feels more affection for the person benefited than the person benefited feels for him."[1]

My criticism of Spencer's explanation is that it does not account for all the phenomena. Indeed, there are some forms of the luxury of pity which it fails to explain —the egoistic pleasure of pity, for example. For it would be a mistake to believe that pity is at all times wholly generous; in fact, it may be attended by very varied egoistic pleasures. To begin with, there may be a feeling of pride, due to an almost unconscious examination of one's own conduct, or a simple feeling of well-being attributable to the vague awakening of the idea of freedom from the misfortunes one is commiserating upon—to the simple effect of contrast. The egoistic sentiment of the man who savours the sweetness of the situation described by Lucretius: "*Suave, mari magno turbantibus æquora ventis,*" *etc.*, is in no way incompatible with a feeling of pity, and dismay at the dangers run. And this is one of the many reasons which enabled La Rochefoucauld to say : "There is in the misfortunes of our best friends something that is not displeasing to us." In these two cases, the compound feeling is less unified than in the analogous case we shall consider later. Again, the 'luxury of pity' is present in persons who take a certain pleasure in feeling kind and compassionate and who relish at their ease the pity which they feel for the woes of other people.

Lastly, in my opinion the pleasure of compassion

[1] *Ibid.*, pp. 625-626.

arises in its purest and most complete form from the tendency to help those we pity, when that tendency is in harmony with most of our ideas or feelings. In all these facts, we observe that multiple effects are produced by the same excitation. That is because the tendency which comes into play and gives rise to so many different feelings is complex and produces different effects according to the tendencies that it calls up in a mind which is itself exceedingly complex. Suppose I am watching an unfortunate person suffer ; on the one hand, the sight tends to oppress me and to make me experience the same kind of suffering ; and, in fact, if the spectacle is very moving, if it hinders the awakening of other feelings, I shall simply experience suffering. But if the representation is not so strong as to dominate consciousness completely, the illusion which tends to be produced tends also to be rectified. Indeed, a representation which does not suspend every activity of the mind is only accepted after having been unconsciously tested by our intelligence ; it agrees or conflicts with our habits of mind and our organized tendencies.

Now if the unhappiness of another be presented to my consciousness without excessive force, it may be inhibited up to a certain point and corrected by a residue of unconscious or almost unconscious reasoning. And then we have, on the one hand, a fairly strong representation of the trouble experienced by another, on the other, a very weak and almost non-existent representation of our own different and relatively better position. In the same way, compassion is at any rate generally accompanied by a tendency to do what we can to help one who is suffering. But if this tendency accords with our personal feelings and our ideas as to the duty of man, it necessarily causes a certain pleasurable feeling. We find further verification of this in the fact that if the tendency to relieve the suffering person is too strongly checked, pity becomes as a rule wholly painful. There is nothing pleasant in seeing someone we love suffer when we are powerless to help ; or at least, if such a feeling is present, it must be due to completely abnormal and pathological causes ; it would be the sign of a peculiar mental perversion and would require other explanations—plurality of psychical systems, reversion to ancestral tendencies, etc.

Similarly, the luxury of grief is further explained by associations of the incipient tendency and the feeling produced with several psychical systems. Quite apart from all the cases in which grief is pleasant, not on its own account, but solely owing to the accessory ideas it recalls, and the case where the pleasure accompanying a painful impression is due to a feeling of pride, it sometimes happens that pain is pleasant, on its own account ; an impression is pleasant because it is unpleasant. This may seem paradoxical. But I believe that it is not so very rare ; and I can state personally that on several occasions a misfortune has given me pleasure by reason of the very annoyance it has induced.

Now let us suppose that we are possessed of general ideas as to the nature of man and the world, morality, duty, æsthetics, and the like, or else of particular ideas as to ourselves or some particular set of circumstances which may arise. Let us suppose that if our theories are correct we ought under such and such conditions to experience a painful impression. If we do not prove to be mistaken, we are then unhappy and satisfied at the same time : unhappy on account of the unpleasantness that occurs, and satisfied because this unpleasantness accords with our expectations and opinions. Sometimes, even, it is not the thing we regard as the objective cause of our grief, but really the grief itself, and that alone, which we find pleasant. This fact, which is illustrated in the ' luxury of pity ', may be observed quite often in persons who reflect upon their feelings ; when, for example, they conclude that their disagreeable impression conforms to the laws of ethics, æsthetics or logic, and that it thus proves the worth of their character.

Thus our general explanation of complex feelings in which pleasure is mingled with pain is that the production of such phenomena involves at the same time a rupture and a consolidation of our mental habits; the process of disorganization which gives rise to pain becomes an element in the general system, and this new organization is productive of pleasure. The concrete explanation varies with each particular case, and also with the nature of the tendencies brought into play. Those which Spencer proposed can be accepted as being of this type. Examples might be multiplied. For instance, a man may be annoyed and displeased at meeting with opposition from a subordinate, and yet this opposition may in certain cases inspire him with respect and on that account be pleasant. Phenomena of this class do not appear to me very difficult to explain with the help of the general law which is simple to apply.

We cannot attempt to review all the compound emotions of this nature. We may, however, relate to the preceding facts several forms of æsthetic pleasure. Thus, the performance of a fine but terrible drama will give us pleasure if the tendencies that arise in us are checked sufficiently early to give us merely the impression of their complexity and their systematization ; but if we do not inhibit them speedily enough, if we go to the length of taking them seriously, we shall experience a mixture of pleasure and pain that may be converted into actual suffering.

Perhaps, in order to have done with this question of pleasant sorrows and painful joys—for we might also consider the latter—we must allow that any restrained activity of the mind, even when it is disagreeable, is capable in certain cases of causing indirectly a certain pleasure.

It may happen that when we read a work written from a point of view entirely opposed to our own we feel a lively admiration for the talent of the author. Here again, a very complex emotion is produced, and for the same reasons as before. On the one hand, the author pleases our literary taste and æsthetic sense ; on the other, he offends our reason. Judging artistically, we are delighted ; judging philosophically, we are displeased. If we endeavour to take everything into consideration at once, we experience a variety of feelings at the same time, such as admiration or respect from one point of view, disapproval, dislike, scorn or indignation from the other. It seems quite clear to me that several very different feelings can be united in this way in a single state of consciousness without entirely combining. The state of consciousness, in this case, is not perfectly definite ; we are 'disquieted', and the various feelings frequently change places with one another and successively dominate consciousness.

Examples could be multiplied ; the law is always the same : different actions are produced when one psychical system is brought into relation with different systems. There is a great multitude of these systems within us, as psychological research and the findings of pathology have shown. What appears to be a very simple fact, the representation of a word, is frequently a system of very diverse elements. It is not astonishing, therefore, if, when a tendency begins to be active, its influence upon these different systems, its conflicts with them, and the different degrees of inhibition which are occasioned at the time, give rise to various affective phenomena, sometimes opposite in character.

We rarely find exact observation and description of these phenomena in scientific works. We ought to find more in literary works, but their validity might be disputed, although, in my opinion, very many of the descriptions are certainly taken from experience. The autobiographies of men of an introspective turn of mind furnish us with valuable information. Take, for example, Rousseau's account of his experiences after his liaison with Madame de Warens had changed in character. We see here all the conditions required for the production of an imperfectly unified complex emotion. Two systems of psychical habits, without any great bond between them, were then of importance in Rousseau's mind. One was that which made him declare that "in order to save me from the perils of youth, it was now time to treat me as a man"—and this concerns the needs which manifest themselves, with some differences, at a certain period in all normally-constituted men ; the other was that which made him address Madame de Warens as 'Mamma', and caused him to say, when speaking of this name, that it expressed very effectively, "the simplicity of our relations, and particularly of our affections." "Never", says Rousseau, "did she dream of withholding her kisses from me, nor the tenderest maternal caresses, and never did it enter into my heart to take advantage of her." And further : "The habit of living a long time innocently together, far from weakening the first sentiments I felt for her, had contributed to strengthen them, giving a more lively, a more tender, but at the same time a less sensual, turn to my affection. Having even accustomed myself to call her 'Mamma', and enjoying the familiarity of a son, it became natural to consider myself as such, and I am inclined to think this was the true reason of my lack of eagerness for the possession of a person I so tenderly loved." Thus the two systems are sufficiently distinct for the experience to be remarkable from the special point of view we are adopting here. Obviously the new relations of Rousseau with his friend were bound to give rise to a very complex state of affairs by acting upon these different systems, and to produce opposite effects and contrary emotions. The mere idea of these relations, once Madame de Warens had informed Rousseau of her intentions, caused a certain disturbance and an appreciable complexity of varying feelings. "I do not know", declares Rousseau, "how to describe the state in which I found myself, filled with a certain dismay mingled with impatience, dreading that which I desired, so much so that at times I earnestly sought in my mind for some worthy means of avoiding my happiness." Finally, here are Rousseau's impressions after Madame de Warens had given herself to him ; they appear to me to confirm completely all that has been stated above :

" The day, more dreaded than hoped for, at length arrived. I promised everything that was required of me, and I kept my word : my heart confirmed my engagement without desiring the prize. I obtained it nevertheless. I found myself for the first time in the arms of a woman—of a woman, too, whom I adored. Was I happy ? No, I tasted pleasure. I know not what invincible sadness empoisoned its relish. It seemed that I had committed an incest, and two or three times, pressing her eagerly in my arms, I deluged her bosom with my tears."[1]

III. *The relatively unified forms of complex affective phenomena*

As the facts of consciousness we have been considering become more and more unified, their complex nature is so much less evident. In cases of violent moral conflict, for example, it is impossible to mistake the complex nature of the feelings experienced ; but when the affective phenomena are relatively well systematized, it becomes more difficult to discern through consciousness the particular nature of the phenomena experienced. Nevertheless, if observation be sufficiently varied, it can very often enlist the aid of induction to distinguish the affective phenomena up to a certain point, and show that their particular tone or *timbre* is due to the encounter and combination of a certain number of different elements. If I employ the word *timbre* in

---

[1] J. J. Rousseau, *Confessions*, Part I, Book V. (*v.* pp. 242-243, English edition, Grant Richards.)

speaking of what gives a feeling its special character, it is because no passion, no feeling, is absolutely the same in different individuals; just as the same note changes in character according as it is emitted by a violin, a flute or a trombone. It seems to me that there is a remarkable analogy between auditory and affective phenomena, and this analogy extends, in my opinion, to all psychical phenomena. In the one case, as in the other, it is a question of a compound impression, which consciousness, unless especially trained, generally perceives as simple; in both cases, this result is probably due to the systematization of impressions, for not every combination of different sounds melts into a single sound, just as not every combination of affective phenomena results in a single affect. In the previous chapter we examined the more or less discordant combinations of affective phenomena; we must now investigate the more harmonious.

In the production of an emotion or a feeling, a considerable part is played by the general condition of the organs and the mind in relation to excitations from without. Often these excitations have merely the effect of liberating in us a certain amount of nervous and mental energy which, according to circumstances, is expended in the awakening of different tendencies. It is a well-known fact that, according to our particular condition, the same things make a pleasant or painful impression, and excite in us very different feelings: love, ambition, hope, fear, etc. I do not wish to dwell upon this here, but rather on the correlative fact of the especial shade, the tone, which the arrival of an excitation from without gives to the feeling already existing in the organism by evoking new tendencies and thus creating new emotive elements.

This case is obviously analogous to those which we studied above, save that there we were dealing with the conflict between the prior state of mind and the phenomena that appeared and created new tendencies, while now we are examining the case in which there is no longer conflict but association.

The fact of systematic association is exceedingly pronounced in violent passions, in overwhelming feelings, when psychical energy is almost entirely absorbed by a single system of tendencies. The impressions which reach the mind through external perception, the tendencies which are thus apt to be awakened, are united and embodied in the general system and, by the admixture of a new element, modify the psychological resultant. The change is, of course, easier to appreciate when it is of some importance.

At other times, the case presents itself differently, but the result, from the point of view of the general psychology of feeling, is absolutely analogous. The tendencies evoked by perception or, in a general way, by a stimulus from the external world or from the organs, become preponderant; but the previous condition of the mind remains and is combined with the newly aroused feeling, to give it a particular *timbre*. Examples of these two classes of facts will, I think, readily occur to the reader. For example, if we have reached a stage of self-confidence and self-satisfaction, slight opposition only makes us feel disdain or pity; if we lack self-confidence, we shall experience anger or discouragement, dejection and a general distaste for the affairs of life; if, combined with pride we have a certain mistrust of the future (feelings by no means mutually exclusive), we shall experience contempt, anger, depression or bitterness, according to the way in which other circumstances, which we cannot attempt to enumerate, present themselves. Circumstances which mingle jealousy, hope or despair with love also provide good material for studying the synthesis of feelings and for seeing how the various tendencies aroused by different causes unite and combine to produce a phenomenon marked by a high degree of unity. We generally notice that a feeling which lasts for some time is as a rule greatly modified under the influence of circumstances, though, for the most part, it retains a certain homogeneity. Some of the tendencies which give rise to it certainly persist all the time the feeling lasts; others change, or cease; others appear again under the pressure of circumstances. It follows that this evolution, which we need not consider in itself, gives rise to a fairly considerable variety of different compounds. The affect changes in character according as its components change; but a certain familiarity with psychological observation is necessary to enable one to perceive the changes and complexity of the phenomenon. In a novel by Tolstoy, *Katia*, there is an interesting study of the changes suffered by love.

As a general rule, it is easy after a little practice to detect the combination of feelings. Unfortunately, these phenomena have been little noted and particular instances and precise facts for quotation are somewhat rare. A great many facts of this kind occur in romance, in poetry, and in all concrete studies of man. A good example of combined feelings, arising from the conjunction of a persistent state of mind with a series of tendencies called up by external perception, is to be found in *Deux Cortèges*, by Joséphin Soulary. The reader can, I think, if he cares to try, find examples of combined sentiments in his own personal experience.

We can doubtless interpret the following observation of Esquirol in this way, and trace the presence of a compound affective phenomenon, produced by the combination of a general habit of mind with a particular impression occurring at certain moments.

"A divisional general, more than fifty years old, had contracted rheumatism during the war, and after a mental affection he became a raging maniac. His teeth were bad and caused him frequent suffering. He accused the sun of being the cause of the troubles he endured; and when the pains were very acute, he uttered terrible cries, abused the sun, and threatened to destroy it with his brave division. Sometimes the pains settled in one knee ; then the patient grasped the painful part with one hand, and closing the other struck great blows upon his knee, repeating 'Ah, villain, you don't escape ! Ah, villain. . . .' He believed that he had a robber in this knee."[1]

Phenomena of this kind may be associated with the well-known fact that all information derived from experience is interpreted in the light of a dominant idea. The phenomena of mental and affective psychology are analogous. We know how often everything in our impressions from the external world which is unrelated to the preoccupations of the mind goes unnoticed by the intelligence. A kind of intellectual selection takes place which allows only the ideas in harmony with the predominant psychical system to pass into consciousness. In the same way, when we are moved by a violent passion, the way in which phenomena are associated is determined almost entirely by the nature of that passion, and all the tendencies and phenomena evoked enter the system of the dominant passion.

But we can witness the creation of compound feelings without the tendencies awakened by an external excitation being combined with tendencies already active in the mind. A tendency which is aroused and which is sufficiently strong to occasion a feeling always excites, as we have seen, a certain number of associated tendencies. Multiplicity of phenomena, which is one of the characteristics of the production of emotion, results from the awakening of certain ill-systematized tendencies, due to various causes (reflex action, dynamogenesis, change in circulation, etc.). It is obvious that these secondary tendencies may also in their turn give rise to affective phenomena. Thus, a powerful feeling such as love is generally accompanied by recollections or images which in their turn establish certain feelings or

[1] Esquirol, *Op. cit.*, I, 209-210.

emotions; and these feelings and emotions blend with the principal feeling and give it a particular colour. A man who is in love may imagine that he is or is not loved; in either case, he may continue to experience the feeling of love. This feeling will always really be love and will have a similar compass, because it is due to the arrest of certain tendencies, to the disturbance of certain psychical systems, which remain the same in both cases; but in each case, the love will have a particular tone: and this particular tone proceeds from the awakening of other tendencies, from the psychical phenomena they bring about, and from the combination in a single state of consciousness of all the psychical elements that tend to be produced by the different systems aroused.

If we briefly consider the complexity of this case, we shall see that the shades are innumerable, even in a single individual, according to the circumstances and to the course that his imagination follows as a consequence of imperceptible influences.

Love is generally accompanied by a certain representation, more or less vague or more or less vivid, of the person loved: this representation may be an image, a sign or an intellectual tendency, but it usually persists in one form or another. The representation does not remain the same; as a general rule we do not limit ourselves to thinking of the object of our love; we imagine the person in particular circumstances—acting and speaking. The actions and words vary entirely in relation to our state of mind, our health, our occupation during the day, the people we have met, the books we have read, the conversations we have had. Then according to the melancholy, sad, cheerful, lascivious, sentimental, tender, excited, or indifferent nature of the image which is called up, and according to the relations of this image with others that are also aroused—the image of the person in a reverie, of a rival, of any individual, of someone unknown—new emotions are produced. We see how prodigious is the variety of shades which a feeling may assume, according as it is accompanied by particular psychical elements due to the evocation of widely differing images and to their combination with others that may differ also.

There are thousands of ways in which a single individual with a moderately active and complex mind may experience the feeling of love. I have only indicated some of them. Other combinations of feeling, which may be produced by different combinations of the imagination, may be taken for granted. Yet the feeling experienced, in spite of its complexity, generally appears as one, and it would be difficult to give direct proof of its complexity, if the variation of circumstance, accompanied by successive variations in feeling, were not so easy to experience and study.

I have spoken of love, because it is one of the strongest and best-known feelings, one of those which most often stimulate the imagination : but any other feeling would serve equally well to establish our point. We should be convinced every time, I believe, that feeling is complex, that it is caused by the excitation of complex tendencies, and that, according to the relations and the degree of systematization of those tendencies, the total affective phenomenon is more or less unified. Pride, ambition, every passion, every feeling that is at all powerful, generally calls up a whole system of tendencies, whose action determines the production of complementary affective phenomena, if I may call them such, which are added to the main impression, and mingled with it, as harmonics combine with a fundamental.

The phenomena which we have reviewed in this chapter have the fairly distinct characteristic of relative co-ordination. It is to this that they owe their greater appearance of unity. We can easily convince ourselves of this by noting the variations of a sentiment: we shall see, I believe, that its unity disappears and its

H

complexity becomes more apparent to consciousness in proportion as the elements are less harmonized and tend to form several unco-ordinated systems. Thus we shall find confirmation of our law by noting how, when a sentiment, or rather the tendencies which produce it, create a tendency or series of tendencies which are separate from and opposed to the first, the subjective unity of the phenomenon disappears at the same time as its unity of co-ordination. So it may come about that love produces jealousy, but the new tendencies that arise in this case can be organized and form a new psychical system : suspicion, mistrust, changing ideas and images, co-ordinated actions, overtures, espionage, and the like. The emotions which arise in this connection are no longer blended with the original feeling ; the feeling which existed in a state of unity first changes, then is broken up and no longer appears simple, even to consciousness. First there was love, then jealous love, then love and jealousy, and sometimes, ultimately, jealousy without love. Here we see the play of tendencies, their complication and their dissociation into two ill-co-ordinated systems, for jealousy is not always compatible with love.

IV. *General analysis. Decomposition of the emotions. Law of compound affective phenomena*

If we continue, from the analytical point of view, the inquiries to which the two last chapters were devoted, we shall be brought to a recognition of the fact that every emotion is a compound emotion, and that the law of its composition is the one we have indicated. But we shall doubtless be able to discover other special laws. There are certain a priori reasons for believing that every affective fact is a compound fact, that every affective phenomenon is due to an arrested tendency and is attended by the awakening of a great number of secondary tendencies. Now, if in the first place

we remember that every conscious event has very complex physiological conditions peculiar to itself, and that
affective phenomena are distinguished from all other
phenomena of consciousness by the complexity of their
conditions and the large number of tendencies whose
evocation is necessary to their production ; and if we
also remember that every tendency is a complex of
psycho-physiological phenomena, we must inevitably
conclude that all affective phenomena, even the weakest,
which we have called signs, are the result of a complex
combination of phenomena.   But we have still to
ascertain the nature of this combination and the relation
of the composite whole to its parts.

We have seen examples of combinations of phenomena in which the elements of an affective state of
consciousness are certainly themselves affects.   Among
these, for instance, are the luxury of pity and the luxury
of grief ; here, in fact, the two different impressions of
pleasure and of pain visibly co-exist in consciousness
with their own characteristics.   This occurs fairly often
in cases of affective phenomena composed of discordant
elements.   These discordant elements, indeed, especially at the beginning when the opposition between them
is most marked, prevent the complete unification of
consciousness ; and, even when the constituent elements
are no longer individually perceptible in the compound,
they are attended by a disturbance of consciousness, by
a sort of oscillation giving rise to a peculiar sensation
to which we shall come back later.

When the constituent affective phenomena of the
total conscious state are sufficiently harmonized, they
are as a rule individually less perceptible.   We can,
however, still distinguish them in many cases—when,
for instance, they are sufficiently intense.   Thus a man
who wants a title or an important position can tell to a
certain extent which elements in his total emotional
state are connected with the power he will be able
to exercise, the social influence his name will give

him, the pleasure of receiving a large salary, and, maybe, the good which his post will enable him to do and the abuses he will be in a position to redress. Each one of the tendencies, which together constitute the representation of his approaching promotion, has a corresponding feeling or a particular affective sign, which modifies, up to a certain point, the emotional whole. And to the total state a new emotion may be added : an æsthetic, moral, egoistic or altruistic emotion, resulting from the contemplation of the functions as a whole, or of their relations to the individual desires or social sentiments of the future official. We have an example of composite feelings whose elements are also affective phenomena and are recognized as such, in the autobiography of John Stuart Mill. He recounts some of the impressions he experienced after the critical period of depression and indifference through which he passed in his youth :

" I at this time first became acquainted with Weber's *Oberon*, and the extreme pleasure which I drew from its delicious melodies did me good by showing me a source of pleasure to which I was as susceptible as ever. The good, however, was much impaired by the thought that the pleasure of music (as is quite true of such pleasure as this was, that of mere tune) fades with familiarity, and requires either to be revived by intermittence, or fed by continual novelty. And it is very characteristic both of my then state, and of the general tone of my mind at this period of my life, that I was seriously tormented by the thought of the exhaustibility of musical combinations. . . . This source of anxiety may, perhaps, be thought to resemble that of the philosophers of Laputa, who feared lest the sun should be burnt out. It was, however, connected with the best feature in my character, and the only good point to be found in my very unromantic and in no way honourable distress." [1]

[1] John Stuart Mill, *Autobiography*, pp. 144-145. Longmans.

Here is another example, taken from Rousseau, who thus analyses his emotions during the performance of *Le Devin du Village*:

" The pleasure of giving emotion to so many amiable persons moved me to tears ; and these I could not contain in the first duo, when I remarked that I was not the only person who wept. . . . I abandoned myself without interruption to the pleasure of enjoying my success. However, I am certain that the voluptuousness of the sex was more predominant than the vanity of the author, and, had none but men been present, I certainly should not have had the incessant desire I felt of catching on my lips the delicious tears I had caused to flow."[1]

Thus, we find that in two very different cases the elements in the compound phenomenon remain distinct. Sometimes the two awakened tendencies are in conflict, sometimes they are in a state of systematic association. Let us examine these two cases : when feelings are in conflict, and appear in the compound with their own characteristics, it is because the opposition is not very keen, and the tendencies to action, or at least one of them, are still very far from being realized. This enables the tendencies and the phenomena they occasion to co-exist without mingling. We must not, in fact, think of consciousness as a sort of narrow field where there is room for only one representation. I can see a red object and a green object at the same time : what I cannot do is to see the same object, at the same time and in the same place, as both red and green. Similarly, I cannot love and hate the same person at the same time for the same reasons and on account of the same qualities ; but I may at the same time, for different reasons and on account of different qualities, both like and dislike him. So long as there is no need for action, so long as the continued existence of the two tendencies does not involve their struggling together to emerge in action

[1] Rousseau, *Confessions*, Part II, Book VIII. (English edition, Vol. II, p. 43.)

or absorb a greater share of psychical energy, the two phenomena produced can co-exist ; and it is precisely because of this want of relationship and this very imperfect systematization that they remain distinct.

But in some cases the elements will remain similarly distinct if they are well enough adapted to one another. The reason here is that one depends on the other. The tendency that produces the second is caused by the tendency that produced the first. The two tendencies, therefore, exist simultaneously, as well as the phenomena to which they give rise ; if now these tendencies occasion different phenomena, such as love and jealousy, for instance, the two phenomena may perfectly well be manifested at the same time. Psychology gives us no reason to expect anything else. Of course, the reverse may also happen, as when, for example, excessive jealousy extinguishes or weakens love ; but we must not at present complicate cases.

We see, then, that in this first case the elements co-exist and persist in the total impression, and that they show themselves fairly distinctly. The total impression is not of appreciable confusion or vagueness. Hence the conditions of this state are : 1, *the difference in the phenomena produced, and the fairly pronounced character of these phenomena ;* 2, *the state of systematization of the tendencies or the lack of relation between them.* The second of these two latter conditions is attended by a sort of partition of consciousness, and the first by an impression of unity.

I will not dwell further on these combinations in which the elements are visibly present with all or nearly all of their characteristics. We have already dealt with a great many instances of them and, besides, they present no difficulty.

We have indirect evidence of the complex nature of feelings and of the part played by the association of the affective phenomena resulting from the excitation of different tendencies, in some of the cases where we are entirely mistaken as to the nature of a feeling we experience. This mistake may be brought about by different causes—sometimes by intellectual and sometimes by affective associations. We will not now go into the question of intellectual associations, which are the conditions of every error; we will merely note that an error in respect of a feeling is not only or always due to the fact that the latter is wrongly classified in the mind, that is to say, that it is systematically associated with ideas or signs which it should not normally excite; for sometimes also it is due to the association of a fundamental tendency with particular tendencies that it ought not logically to arouse and whose nature causes us to be mistaken as to the nature of the principal tendency. Here the intellectual association which constitutes the error is secondary and not primary; it is determined by the grouping of affective phenomena. Thus we often think that we are acting on very lofty impulses, when actually our motives are of a very commonplace order. The superior tendency is excited secondarily and has scarcely any power, but for reasons easy to understand it is associated more closely with the intellectual phenomena while the fundamental tone is hardly perceived by consciousness. We have here a complex affective phenomenon in which one element attracts the greater part of the attention, so that the mind, by failing to consider the others sufficiently, is mistaken as to the nature of the phenomenon as a whole. Facts of this description are well known; and man is usually very ingenious in making virtues of his defects, by ignoring many of the phenomena aroused by the tendencies which have impelled him to action.

When it was proposed to present Rousseau to the king, after the performance of *Le Devin du Village*, and the prospect of a pension was held out to him, Rousseau refused and departed.

He explains his reasons in this way: "My first idea . . . was concerned with my frequently wanting to retire; this had made me suffer very considerably at the theatre and might torment me the next day when I should be in the gallery, or in the King's apartment, amongst all the great, waiting for His Majesty to pass. This infirmity was the principal cause which prevented me from mixing in polite companies, and shutting myself up in female society. The idea alone of the situation in which this want might place me was sufficient to produce it to such a degree as to make me feel sick, if I would not adopt a mode of relief to which death was preferable in my eyes. None but persons who are aquainted with this situation can judge of the horror which being exposed to the risk of it inspires. "I then supposed myself before the King, presented to his Majesty, who deigned to stop and speak to me. In this situation justness of expression and presence of mind were peculiarly necessary in answering. Would my accursed timidity, which disconcerts me in the presence of any stranger whatever, have been shaken off in the presence of the King of France, or would it have suffered me instantly to make choice of proper expressions? . . . What, said I, will become of me in this moment, and before the whole Court, if, in my confusion, one of my usual ill-timed phrases should escape me? This danger alarmed and terrified me ; I trembled to such a degree that at all events I was determined not to expose myself to it.

"I was thus losing, it is true, the pension which in some measure was offered to me, but I was at the same time exempting myself from the yoke it would have imposed. Adieu truth, liberty and courage. How should I afterwards have dared to speak of disinterested-ness and independence? Had I received the pension, I must either have become a flatterer or remained silent ; and, moreover, who would have insured to me the pay-ment of it? What steps should I have been under the necessity of taking? How many people must I have solicited ! I should have had more trouble and anxious cares in preserving than in doing without it. Therefore,

I thought I acted according to my principles by refusing, and sacrificing appearance to reality."[1]

We can see from this how complex must have been the composite state of mind preceding Rousseau's decision. He, as a matter of fact, seems to be aware of all the factors, but many in his position would, I think, as Rousseau himself often did, have misinterpreted their feelings and have attributed to a noble love of independence, not merely that share of influence which was its due, but also that which was induced by other considerations of a perfectly defensible but obviously inferior nature. If it were not outside the scope of our present inquiry, this would be the place to show how commonplace or even reprehensible feelings can give rise to higher feelings and how the tendencies are engendered and strengthened or supplanted.

It frequently happens that the component phenomena almost disappear, or at least are difficult to perceive. Here again, in order to explain the phenomenon which is then produced, I shall take analogies from the laws of perception and try to justify them. It is not very surprising that such analogies do exist, since all psychical facts are subject to general laws which are manifested in an analogous manner through various classes of phenomena. The following experiment can easily be made with the aid of a stereoscope, or simply with a piece of cardboard. Look at a rectangle of blue paper with one eye, and a rectangle of red paper with the other, and then attempt to superpose the two images. The resulting image is hazy and shifting, sometimes inclining to blue, sometimes to red, sometimes violet— vague and ill-defined. If white and black paper are used instead of coloured papers, we know that a sensation of dazzle is experienced, resulting from the unequal luminous excitation received by the two eyes. So with affective phenomena it seems to me that a kind of vague,

---

[1] Rousseau, *Confessions*, Part II, Book VIII. (English edition, Vol. II, pp. 44-45.)

confused, ill-defined compound is produced, which is strikingly analogous to this dazzle. It is chiefly produced when I think of persons whose character and intelligence please me in certain respects while they displease me in others. The phenomenon is especially marked, of course, when I think of the person as a whole; when I dwell exclusively upon particular qualities in him, my impression becomes much clearer; but it becomes a little confused again if my attention is not closely concentrated on account of associations which cannot be entirely eliminated.

But when I am most favourably placed for observing the phenomenon, my impression wavers; sometimes one feeling prevails, sometimes the other, or a combination is formed; the two opposite impressions cancel each other out. Most frequently, the phenomenon is not sufficiently differentiated; its elements remain in the penumbra of consciousness, unless attention calls them forth, and the compound gives only a vague and blurred impression. The various psychical systems that have come into operation cannot be co-ordinated or supplanted: one of them prevails for a moment, and impresses itself upon consciousness, but a sudden change soon takes place. The phenomenon is accentuated, perhaps, and displays itself in a clearer form if we have to perform an action which concerns the person whose character makes these various impressions upon us; if, for instance, we have the opportunity of doing him a service, and have a good excuse for ignoring it. The oscillation of the phenomena will be shown by the oscillation of the will and by the contradictory character of the inclinations that assert themselves. Further, if we decide to render or refuse the service, that is to say, if one of the two psychical systems be completed by the bringing into play of the appropriate muscles, the other system does not absolutely cease to function, and will be manifested affectively by dissatisfaction and regret.

It is very difficult to describe exactly that particular state of disturbance which I venture to call the *affective lustre*. It resembles, however, in many respects the synthetic perception that results from the simultaneous perception of white and black, or of two different colours, while at the same time it is in many ways different. Nevertheless, I think sufficient has been said for the reader to remember his own experiences of this condition, and to be able to recognize it.

What are the conditions of this phenomenon? Apart from the general conditions of affective facts, it seems to me that their special characteristics can be referred to *the simultaneous or almost simultaneous coming into play* [1] *of systems which tend towards opposite or different actions and which cannot both culminate in action at the same time; always provided that the psychical systems brought into play do not differ too widely in intensity, and that their opposition is at least beginning to manifest itself.*

In fact, here we see the differences between this case and the preceding one. The mind being a complex of psychical systems, several of these may be in activity without any opposition being exhibited among them, if they occasion different actions which can be performed at the same time, and if none of them absorbs too great a share of psychical energy. These systems may actually function or begin to function in a sufficiently active and violent manner to occasion consciousness and even affective phenomena. We have seen instances of this. But if each of these systems tends to express itself in different actions which cannot be performed at the same

---

[1] A complete simultaneity of very distinct psychical manifestations of opposite systems of tendencies is not absolutely necessary, because, in all the cases that we have seen, when the psychical phenomena follow one another rapidly with no quite obvious form of co-existence, the psycho-physiological activity which produced them does not absolutely cease and shows itself by less apparent phenomena—by affective and intellectual signs, which suffice to impart to the new phenomenon, produced by the coming into play of the opposite system, a particular character of complexity.

time, a compound results, that is more unified—*i.e.* its elements are less apparent—but less distinct and more confused, especially if these opposed psychical systems are linked together and activated by the same external impressions, or by the same images. If other analogies from the field of perception be required, they will be found in sound dissonance, and particularly in beats.

But in some cases the elements in the affective phenomenon become still less evident. It is well known that an untrained ear is entirely unable to distinguish the parts played by each instrument in an orchestra, and does not even know what instruments are combining in the general effect. That does not prevent the whole impression, however simple it may appear to consciousness, from being composed of particular impressions, and varying according to the variations of the particular impressions, even though the latter are not individually perceived. Even in a consonance it is difficult or impossible for many persons to distinguish the elements in the total effect, yet these elements are perceived by consciousness, and their slightest variations produce a very clear impression ; none the less, a consonance appears as a simple sound. Moreover, a musical sound is generally a harmony whose elements are not separately perceived, and yet they are clearly manifest to consciousness, since a change in them is shown by an alteration in the *timbre* of the sound. In the same way, we find affective phenomena composed of affective elements which are imperceptible and not recognized by consciousness as such.

Here we are confronted by an important question, which must not be evaded. It may be asked whether a similar decomposition of the sensations or feelings into their psychical elements is an entirely justifiable operation; and whether, indeed, it has any relevant interpretation. I will try to state the objection in its full force : when we hear a sound or experience a feeling the total state of consciousness is the synthesis of several perceptions or of several affective phenomena. But introspection reveals nothing of this. I am conscious of a single sound or a single feeling, which does not seem to me to be compound; but sensations, however elementary they may be, and psychical phenomena, however rudimentary we may think them, appear to be capable of existing only so long as they are present to consciousness. If, however, in spite of appearances, the sensation or the feeling be composed of psychical elements, sensational or emotional, these sensations and emotions are not perceived by consciousness: which appears contradictory. Can an emotion or a sensation have any possible existence if it is not perceived as such by consciousness?

The difficulty will disappear, I believe, when we show that it is simply based on an ambiguity. The word consciousness has, unfortunately, more than one meaning. Apart from the confusion between psychological consciousness and moral consciousness or conscience, and confining ourselves entirely to the former, the word sometimes denotes the most abstract general quality of subjective phenomena and at other times it has almost the signification of knowledge. Thus, we call a tendency unconscious when it is unaccompanied by a clear idea of its object, even although it may be manifested by the emotions, as, for example, the sexual tendency, when it begins to appear in subjects who are ignorant of its nature. Yet this may be a misuse of terms, and, if we are not on our guard against the possible double signification of the word, a cause of error. It may very well be maintained, moreover, that such tendencies are completely conscious, though unrecognized and unclassified. And it is clear that the risk of changing from one meaning to another in the course of an argument inevitably involves a danger of erroneous and contradictory conclusions.

In point of fact, I believe that what we ought to say

is that in a compound sound, a piano-note, we are conscious of all the component sounds, as sounds; but the intellectual phenomena which generally accompany the sensation of sound, and assist in its classification, do not in this case accompany the sensation of every sound, but only the sensation of the whole. As we know, indeed, a perception is a very complex phenomenon, a mixture of intellectual and sensorial activity; every sensation, on reaching the brain, is recognized, interpreted and classified; and it is with these various modifications that we perceive it. In the case of compound perception, not each individual sensation is classified and interpreted, but the whole which they form. The elementary sensations are deprived of their intellectual associations, and consequently they are unrecognized—we will not say by consciousness, which registers but does not recognize—but by the intelligence. They are none the less existent as psychical elements, since consciousness registers the change introduced by each of them; and, taken separately, they give rise to very clear states of consciousness. They exist, then, as facts of consciousness, but not as intellectual facts.

They may, of course, acquire the latter quality. Doubtless this changes the phenomenon, and the psychical element is no longer what it was before. But this difference, as experience seems to show, in no way affects the psychical character of the phenomenon, but rather the character which its complete classification gives to it. We can test this by learning to distinguish the harmonics which make up a fundamental tone. I myself am able to distinguish the fifth most readily. This clearer perception does not appear to me to modify sensibly the subjective character of the sound; there is merely greater distinctness in the perception of the element that chiefly occupies my attention. Similarly, to recognize a perfect chord, and to distinguish the three notes which compose it, does not change the total effect to any considerable extent. There is no new sensation, but simply a recognition of, and a distinction between, sensations which existed before as phenomena of consciousness, without being known or rigorously classified. I do not wish to suggest that they were completely unclassified, for it would appear that every psychical fact, by reason of the systematization of our organs and established associations, must be to some extent classified and systematized; but it will be understood that this classification may be more or less definite and complicated, and that the associations of a fact with the group of tendencies constituting the ego may be more or less numerous and more or less organized.

Similarly, in my opinion, we find in complex feelings psychical elements which are not recognized and yet are also affective elements. There are the same reasons for admitting this as there were for admitting that sensations may be combined in a complex perception, to all appearance one, without thereby ceasing to exist in themselves as phenomena of consciousness.

It is chiefly in sufficiently unified affective states that the phenomenon of harmonious complexity is to be observed. And it is also necessary, as we saw, that these psychical elements should not engross the attention, either by their intensity or by any peculiar characteristic whatsoever. We know, in fact, that for a psychical compound to appear simple individual constituent elements must not be strongly united with other phenomena and other tendencies. In a word, they must be more closely associated among themselves than with other facts; and the ensemble alone must have preponderant importance in the psychological mechanism. We see here the dissociation and recomposition of phenomena described in the statement of the principles of general psychology given in the first part of this work. Individual component factors lose all their psychical associations, except those that connect them with the other elements of the same system.

When we gaze at a monument some distance away,

so that we can see the whole of it without being too far removed to note the details, we undoubtedly see those details and our perceptions of them certainly exist in us as facts of consciousness; but we can very easily not notice them, and devote our attention to the monument as a whole. Nevertheless, this perception of the whole is not unattended by consciousness—I do not say knowledge of the details. At this moment, the details are not connected by any association with our tendencies, our emotions, or our ideas; they are merely associated to form the whole, and it is that whole, as such, which is the object of our reflections or our feelings. Yet even while remaining conscious of the whole, we may notice some detail more particularly, that is to say, we may associate it more strongly and more definitely with the other phenomena of the ego. We see that the conception of the whole remains much the same.

Passing to affective facts, we may observe a similar state of affairs. But one circumstance which frequently prevents the component elements from being clearly distinguished is that some, from their very nature, are difficult to perceive distinctly—affective impulses, for example, and affective signs. The result is that affective phenomena of a high order are not easy to resolve into their affective elements. These affective elements are aroused by the arrest of tendencies whose existence sometimes is only then revealed to us by the affective phenomena they cause. Hence, it is a very delicate matter to analyse in detail the elements of the phenomenon, even apart from the difficulty which is presented by the resolution of a fact which we are accustomed to regard as a whole and not in its constituent elements.

A partial analysis, however, is not impossible, even for the higher feelings. In the friendship or esteem which we feel for a particular person at a particular moment, we can certainly distinguish as separate elements the impression which some action of his or the reading of one of his works has produced in us. In the admiration we feel for the genius of a writer, it is obviously possible to distinguish the impression which was made upon us by some particular page of his works or some particular quality of his imagination, intelligence, or style. In love, one is generally able to observe the impression caused by some special qualities of the person loved, or by some special event in which he or she has taken part. We can thus ascertain the place which the rise of a particular tendency occupies in the total phenomenon.

A good method of analysing feeling is to notice that even the abstract images and ideas which accompany it have all a fairly strong affective colouring, and that this affective colouring accompanies ideas that are represented to consciousness only by very vague abstract signs. If I attempt to revive the impression of a certain country walk, for instance, I see vague, abstract, colourless images rising before me. At the same time, a certain number of affective phenomena connected with these images appear and become harmonized. Thus, although consciousness is seldom occupied by more than one image, other images, and ideas associated with them, still manifest themselves by abstract signs, accompanied by affective phenomena which may be more or less powerful. I think an example of analysis and decomposition of feeling may be seen in the following passages from the second letter of Héloïse to Abélard. Unfortunately psychological phenomena are never described with sufficient minuteness or precision to enable us directly to observe and ascertain the facts ; we are reduced to interpreting them, to reconstituting the psychological state, and to conjecturing it in a certain measure ; nevertheless, I am probably not mistaken in seeing in the following lines indications of phenomena such as I have described—a passion in which we meet with particular affective elements, co-operating to produce the whole, and associated with images or intellectual signs : " . . . hæc quidem amaritudo veræ poenitentiæ quam rara sit Beatus diligenter attendens Ambrosius : ‘ Facilius ’, inquit, ‘ inveni qui innocentiam servaverunt quam qui poenitentiam egerunt.’ In tantum vero illæ quas pariter exercuimus, amantium voluptates dulces mihi fuerunt at nec displicere mihi, nec vix a memoria labi possint. Quocunque loco me vertam semper se oculis meis cum suis ingerunt desideriis ; nec etiam dormienti suis illusionibus parcunt. Inter ipsa Missarum solemnia, ubi purior esse debet oratio, obscæna earum voluptatum fantasmata ita sibi penitus miserrimam captivant animam, ut turpitudinibus illis magis quam orationi vacem. Quæ cum ingemiscere debeam de commissis, suspiro potius de amissis. Nec solum quæ egimus, sed loca pariter et tempora in quibus hæc egimus, ita tecum nostro infixa sunt animo, ut in ipsis omnia tecum agam, nec dormiens etiam ab his quiescam. Nonnunquam et ipso motu corporis animi mei cogitationes deprehenduntur, nec a verbis temperant improvisis.” [1]

(. . . Considering diligently how rare is this severity of true penitence, the Blessed Ambrose declares : ‘ More easily have I found those who have preserved their innocence, than those who have exercised penitence.’ Such, indeed, in a like manner, were for me those dear delights of lovers, in which we engaged, as neither to displease me, nor to pass from my recollection. Whithersoever I turn, they thrust themselves, with longings, before my eyes ; during sleep itself, I am not spared visions of them. Even during the solemn rites of Masses, when prayer should be more free from impurity, the immodest apparitions of those pleasures seek to entrap for themselves my most miserable soul, so that I may occupy myself more with such shamefulness than with prayer. When I ought to groan at having committed them, I more readily sigh at having left them behind. Not only what we did, but also the places where we practised those things, and the times

[1] *Magistri Petri Abelardi et Heloissæ epistolæ*, p. 59.

when we practised them, are with thyself so imprinted on my soul, that there and then I do with thee all things, neither do I forbear from them, even while sleeping. Sometimes, indeed, the meditations of my soul are captured by the very movement of my body, nor do they abstain from unconsidered words.)

In a general way, the purely sensual side, the more emotional aspect—the intellectual feeling, so to speak—may be fairly easily recognized in the feeling of love and in passion.

Again, the complex character of feelings is most clearly revealed by the change they undergo, so long as that change does not pass unnoticed by the person experiencing the feelings. Thus we feel our admiration for an author increase or diminish after reading a new work he has written. The psychical element stirred up by the latter circumstance is amalgamated with the others, but it can still be discerned in the combination.

The complete analysis of a feeling, however, remains almost always impossible, for the reasons we have stated. The elements are too difficult to disentangle. An additional circumstance which prevents our entering further on the subject is that the elements which combine to form a compound affective phenomenon are not all phenomena of the affective class ; and we shall have to revert to the point in relation to this new form of synthesis. In affective phenomena where the elements are less complex, it is easier to disentangle the elementary parts whose systematization forms the total impression. In the pleasure from the affective sensation we receive from an elaborate dish, for example, it is still difficult to ascertain the particular pleasure caused by the perception of each element, though it is sometimes possible. The pleasure afforded by the smell of truffles, for instance, is an easily recognizable fact, and on the other hand, by cutting out certain ingredients the dish as a whole may be so altered that we know very definitely what is wanting ; a lack

of salt, for example, is readily noticed. Numerous
instances of this kind could, I think, be cited.

Nevertheless, when we have resolved a feeling into
its constituent elements, we have not explained it.
Even when detailed analysis has revealed to us all the
psychical elements of some emotion, passion, or other
complex phenomenon, we cannot reconstruct the whole
from them, for the very simple reason that there is a
part of the compound which cannot be discovered in its
concrete elements, I mean the composition itself and the
relation of the parts to each other. The impression
made upon us by a monument is not the sum of the
impressions which would be aroused in us by the sum
of the stones used in its construction. If we ate, one
after another, all the elements which enter into the
composition of an excellent dish, we should certainly
not always experience a pleasant impression. Similarly, the admiration we feel for a beautiful statue is not
to be equated with our admiration for the head, plus our
admiration for the arms, plus our admiration for the
torso, etc. In short, there is in every compound which
is not a mere juxtaposition of heterogeneous parts
(and this would be true even in that case) something
which cannot be traced in the components. A systematized feeling is not a sum of feelings, but a feeling at
once single and complex, enveloping and binding
together secondary feelings.

There are cases in which this distinction between the
whole and the parts is especially noteworthy : in these,
the relation between the components gives rise to a
compound characterized by an affective colouring not
possessed by the elements. We saw numerous examples
when speaking of ill-systematized emotions, such as the
impression of agitation and conflict which attends the
simultaneous production of two contrary emotions. In
that case, the elements still exist, but their relations are
made manifest by a phenomenon that is evident and
separable by analysis from either component. Even

when the result of the relationship is not so exactly observable, all the analogies plead in favour of its existence; the very existence of the union of the elements in one and the same state of consciousness indicates relations between them, and that those relations enter also as elements into the total composition of the phenomenon, experiment and induction do not permit us to doubt. We see, consequently, that the decomposition of affective phenomena and, I would add, of all complex phenomena, is perfectly legitimate and leads to results. Nevertheless, we are unable to discover in the isolated parts all that is found in the whole; and, in order to explain the latter, a great deal of attention must be paid to the relations of the components.

Furthermore, it is only by the relations of the parts that it is possible to explain the analysis in the case where the elements are not phenomena of the same order as the compound. We have seen the conditions of the appearance of affective phenomena; we noticed that those conditions, the rise and arrest of tendencies, multiplicity of phenomena, relative inco-ordination, sudden appearance, etc., are very complex, and that, according as one or other of them varies in intensity, or is altogether absent, the nature of the affective phenomenon is changed. We are concerned here with a resultant of a different order from the phenomena which have produced it; and it is with reference to facts of this kind that psychical combinations have been compared with chemical combinations, where the compound is very different from its constituents. In the examples which we are examining, however, the case is not absolutely the same. In fact, when an emotion is produced under the conditions we have indicated, the phenomena that are the conditions of the production do not disappear. The emotion does not absorb them; it emerges from them, so to speak; it results from the relations of the phenomena thus produced to the character and general habits of the organism. The most probable hypothesis as to its formation and nature is that it is the general correlative of all the particular phenomena which are then produced, and of the relations of these phenomena with the persistent tendencies of the mind, whilst all these phenomena, or at least many of them, possess at the same time their special psychical correlatives. Thus, when we experience a sufficiently powerful feeling, we distinctly feel the beating of our heart, the quickening or slackening of our breathing and all the other detailed phenomena that are then produced, such as images, ideas, etc. We undoubtedly have a certain consciousness, if not a clear and considered knowledge of them, but the emotion is not any one of these details, nor is it their sum : it appears to be the psychical impression of the relations of all the particular phenomena among themselves and with the organized tendencies which are more or less affected by them. Emotion, feeling, every affective phenomenon in general would thus be a sort of psychological synthesis of various elements, which themselves belong to the class of affective phenomena or to other classes.

Our reason for adopting this point of view is that we see emotions behaving in the presence of the diverse conditions which we have enumerated as a resultant behaves towards the phenomena that produce it : varying with them, appearing, disappearing, augmenting or decreasing in intensity under certain appreciable conditions, according as its factors vary, appear, disappear, increase or diminish.[1] I tried to give proofs of this in the first part of this study, by means of observation, analysis, and synthesis.

Moreover, there does not seem to be anything very

---

[1] I realize, nevertheless, that this argument is not sufficient to ensure the acceptance of the hypothesis I propose. Other likely hypotheses may be advanced : suppose, for example, that the affective phenomenon is not the psychological correlative of the numerous physiological phenomena then produced, but simply of one of the physiological phenomena which resulted from the others. The best course, in my opinion, is to reserve judgment.

mysterious in the fact that elements of a particular character should condition a fact of a different character. Insistence upon the necessity for discovering in the cause the qualities of the effect, which is still sometimes put forward as a rule of logic, is based on a hollow sophism, which some would like to make into an axiom. I see no necessity for admitting that "everything which is present in an effect ought to be present in the cause". Indeed, that can only rest upon a metaphysical conception of cause ; and further, it might be maintained that the metaphysical theory of cause in no way implies the truth of the traditional axiom. But I would ask those who hold that cause is an assemblage of conditions, and that the only things we need look for are phenomena and the relations between them, why we should discover in a phenomenon the qualities that are present in the phenomena with which it is connected by a law ? There is no good reason for this, and the axiom has been established by superficial analogies.

The study of the composition and decomposition of feelings has led us to admit that the relations of various mental tendencies and various psychical systems are the cause of the particular facts that give a complex character to an affective phenomenon. We have seen that the awakening of various ideas, various tendencies, everything, in short, which happens to modify the circumstances of the production of a feeling, also modifies the feeling itself. The compound changes with its elements. But, in different persons, or in the same person at different times, associations between psychical phenomena take place in different ways ; everything is a little different—physical nature and psychical nature, the habits of the organs of vegetative life, and the habits of the organs of mental life. The psychical systems are different, and differently combined. Thus, when a closely analogous tendency is excited by closely analogous influences, the train of concomitant phenomena differs greatly in different persons, or in the same person at different times, although the differences are generally less obvious in the latter case, provided the periods are not too far apart. Likewise, feelings, emotions and all affective phenomena differ enormously in different persons. Every emotion, every passion, bears the mark of the personality in whom it appears. It afterwards reacts upon that personality, which, however, it can modify only by imposing itself; that is to say, by generating a complex of phenomena which is in fact the physiological concomitant of the affective phenomenon. Not that every affective phenomenon affects the entire personality, but it affects at least some psychical systems which are never again the same. There are no two similar emotions; love according to John Stuart Mill is not the same as love according to Casanova. Similarly, the same man is not usually amorous, or ambitious, or proud at forty in exactly the same way as at eighteen. These are well-known facts, upon which I need not insist. It is often possible to refer these various types of feeling to general causes of which sex is one. If we consider, for example, the passion of sensual love, in nymphomaniacs and in sexual maniacs, we observe a remarkable difference in the colouring and *timbre* of this passion, and the difference is shown in the means adopted to gratify it.

In illustration of what I term the harmonic tones of passion, and the modifications that they cause in the fundamental tone: " We must emphasize here ", says Legrand du Saulle, "an important difference, which the majority of authors have noted, between the conduct and habits of nymphomaniacs and sexual maniacs. Both bring into play, in the unrestrained pursuit of sexual gratification, the tendencies peculiar to their sex. The man is often brutal and violent; he rushes at the first woman he meets, and does not allow her to resist him. Should she not yield to his desires, he will beat her, forcibly violate her, and sometimes even kill

her. The woman has recourse rather to the charm of
her manners and to coquetry ; she omits none of the
means of seduction that are in her power, but she never
uses brutality or violence : at the most, she will respond
with irony and abuse to the indifference that offends
her and the contempt that distresses her. We have an
example of a satyriasiac in Léger, who was condemned
to death in 1824 at the Assizes of Seine-et-Oise for
kidnapping and violating a young girl, and feeding on
her blood, after killing her. An instance of nympho-
mania is found in the woman mentioned by Marc, who
induced the man upon whom she had fixed her regard
" to enjoy a bath with her ", and again in the woman
described by Buisson, who eyed men brazenly, solicited
the first comer, and if scorned became furious and
abusive, adopting an attitude of sarcastic contempt."[1]

Again, we find a general modification of feeling in
certain diseases : it is known that epilepsy, general
paralysis and phthisis give a certain general colour,
nearly always the same, to affective phenomena. Finally,
there remains physiological make-up, what we call temperament. The science of temperaments is far from
being established; physiology has not supplied sufficient
indications in reference to these matters to justify
psychology in building up doubtful theories. "The doctrine of temperaments ", says Ribot, "old as medicine
itself, always criticized and always being restated, is
the vague and fluctuating expression of the principal
types of physical personality, as shown by observation,
together with the principal psychical characteristics
which spring from them. . . . If the determination of
temperaments could become scientific, the problem of
personality would be greatly simplified."[2] I shall not,
therefore, attempt to draw up a psychological classification of temperaments. Such an attempt will be found
at the end of the *Physiologie des passions* by Letourneau

---

[1] Legrand du Saulle, " Les Nymphomanes ", *Les Hystériques*, p. 603.
[2] Ribot, *Les Maladies de la personnalité*, p. 29.

who has tried to revive the old formulæ and bring them into stricter accordance with actual facts. I shall confine myself, for the moment, to pointing out the general influence of personality on the production of feeling, an influence of which, moreover, we have had numerous examples. Considerations relating to associations of conscious phenomena and to the influences that feeling exercises, or to which it is subject, belong rather to the study of the laws of the evolution and organization of phenomena than to that of their appearance.

The decomposition of the emotions and the laws that govern the appearance of complex affective phenomena enable us to observe various applications of the general law stated in the first chapter. What we have tried to do is to refer the composition of the emotions to the general phenomena which we saw in the production of each affective phenomenon, by showing what method of grouping and association, what particular aspect of the general conditions of emotion gave rise to particular compound affective phenomena. Thus we have successively seen the part played by the arrest of tendencies, and the counter-arrest of tendencies which arrest those just activated ; the association and conflict of psychical phenomena and psychical systems ; the strife and incoordination of phenomena, the multiplicity of secondary psychical and physical phenomena, etc. I would now sum up the theories to which we have been led and formulate the general laws governing the appearance of compound affective phenomena in the following manner.

The subjective character of unity of a compound affective phenomenon is proportionate to the systematization of the tendencies which excite the relatively simple affective phenomena co-existing in a state of consciousness. Two or more feelings may be awakened at the same time by the simultaneous activation of several psychical systems. According as these psychical systems remain active for some time without entering into direct relations or without one of them tending to check the activity of the other, or according as they form a new association which brings them together in a higher system, the two affects either subsist in isolation without giving rise to a synthetic compound, or else produce a complex phenomenon in which the elements subsist but which is accompanied by a new synthetic affective phenomenon, resulting from the relations between component phenomena. If there is conflict between the partial systems, the compound phenomenon will be characterized by disturbance, oscillation, vibration, comparable in some respects to the vibrations of discordant sounds, or with the perception of lustre : if there is association, the compound phenomenon possesses such a decided character of unity that its analysis by direct observation becomes relatively difficult, and slight emotions, faint accessory feelings, are combined with the principal, like harmonics with their fundamental tone. The variation according to persons and times in the combination of elementary affective phenomena explains in great measure their correlative difference and makes them an incomplete but important expression of personality.

CONCLUSION

I DESIRE in conclusion to consider briefly the conditions of the appearance of affective phenomena from the synthetic standpoint of general psychology. Man, as we have said before, is an assemblage of innumerable elements, bound up in many systems in such a manner that the same element can successively enter a great number of systems, which are themselves elements in still larger systems; and so on, until we come to the personality regarded as a whole, which should be the greatest system of all, if man's organization were complete; but it presents a remarkable incoherence, so that the secondary systems are not united in a superior system, and instead of joining and combining they often interfere with one another. This assemblage of systems, which is man, is in relation with the outer world; the impressions, which reach him from it, are organized within him, decomposed and recomposed. The inner mechanism receives and assimilates these, first analysing and then synthesizing them; man being a kind of machine, which dissociates the combinations that present themselves simultaneously in space and time, and, from the elements thus obtained, makes new associations, determined by the relations of the facts among themselves and with the previously acquired organization which by assimilation they help to form. Furthermore, these systems in man are composed of various elements. Some are received from outside whilst others return there; systems of sensations and ideas lead to systems of movements, and both are organized together. So we picture man as a sort of imperfectly finished or somewhat disordered machine, which, receiving impressions from without, decomposes and synthesizes them by combinations of numerous internal cog wheels, and so reacts as to augment in a certain measure the systematization of the outside world simultaneously with its own.

From all that we have said with regard to the appearance of affective phenomena, it is evident that they are the sign of a violent disturbance of the organism, an imperfect functioning of the machine. They appear when the systematic reaction of the organism is impeded, when nervous energy, liberated by an external or internal excitation, cannot be turned to a useful purpose, when neither harmony of internal tendencies nor harmony of action can be obtained. On this account, and for similar reasons, every conscious event is an indication of a disturbance of the organism, affective phenomena pointing to a disturbance more considerable than that which is indicated by other conscious events. Every passion, every emotion, every feeling, is therefore the sign of an imperfection in the organism.

This conclusion clearly emerges from all the circumstances accompanying the production of emotion; all the circumstances which we studied in the first chapter —the arrest of tendencies, the rush of blood to the brain, the rise in temperature, the multiplicity of phenomena, their relative inco-ordination, etc.—must be interpreted in this sense. In classifying them from the point of view of synthetic psychology, we find that they can be referred to three main facts: the rise of psychical or psycho-organic systems, or parts of systems, imperfectly co-ordinated with the dominant tendency; a lack of co-ordination among elements or systems brought into play simultaneously and possessed of equal importance; and lastly, a lack of certain psychical elements necessary to the harmonious functioning of the mind. These phenomena must be fairly pronounced to give rise to an affect; they are always a consequence of the primary fact which we have shown to be the bringing into play of a relatively considerable psychical force which cannot be harmoniously employed.

Instead of continuing from this point of view the examination of the various affective phenomena and the facts that produce or accompany them, a study which does not seem to me to present any serious difficulty, I shall confine myself to indicating how these laws operate in certain circumstances.

The first case presents itself when, for instance, the association of psychical elements with a view to action is not effected without some disturbance, that is to say, without the calling up of other elements which are associated with the first and which ought not to be aroused in these circumstances. An example will help to make my meaning clear. Let us suppose that a surgeon, when performing an operation, is moved by the thought of the pain he is causing his patient, the risks involved by the operation, or the distress of the patient's family. The feeling which results from the relations of the images of all these phenomena with his own actions clearly shows us that associated with the system of psychical elements set in activity in order to perform the operation are certain elements which form part of other systems, which ought not to have been called up at that moment; these elements being the idea of the family's grief, the patient's suffering, etc. Now, these images, these ideas, or these signs, are closely associated with the sight of a suffering man ; but such associations cannot enter into the psychical system which must control the operation. Thus we see here associations which have not been completely severed and whose elements are not dynamically isolated in such a way as to allow one to be evoked without involving the evocation of the others, so that each can enter separately into different psychical combinations. This fact, resulting from the excessive cohesion of the elements of phenomena and from the difficulty of dissociation which would permit them to enter into different psychical systems, while preserving the cohesion necessary to enable them in case of need to form part of the same system, is one of the great causes of the psychical disturbance which produces affective phenomena. It is very frequently encountered, and can be discerned in a large number of the examples we have given.

Another cause is the difficulty of association sometimes experienced in co-ordinating elements when some of them are outside the range of association of the tendencies whose systematization they would promote. This is the case, for instance, when we desire to grasp the relations of several facts, and the operation becomes sufficiently difficult to give rise to an affective phenomenon.

One more cause, finally, is the absence of appropriate psychical elements, which may occur, for example, in emotions which are accompanied by desire ; the actions towards which the system whose activity gives rise to them tends, are, as a rule, aimed directly at supplying the missing elements.

The difficulty is increased again in the simultaneous activation of two psychical systems which would naturally culminate in actions which cannot be performed at the same time.

Thus, difficulty of association, difficulty of dissociation, and the lack of elements necessary to fulfil a tendency, are the principal causes which fall under the general heading of obstacles to the systematization of the organism and the mind. These are the general characteristics of affective phenomena from the standpoint of general psychology.

The theory which sees in activity merely a manifestation of a profound disturbance of the personality is, or appears to be, in contradiction to the most widely prevailing views. We are accustomed to regard sensibility as a quality indicating by its presence a superior personality. To appraise the relative value of the various factors of human personality is the business of ethics. Here I will say only a few words to indicate the causes which explain, and in some measure justify, current opinion. It may be affirmed in a general way that many characteristics which would be defects in relation to a very advanced state of development, are good qualities in relation to the actual condition of man. Feeling, in the psychological sense, is one of these characteristics; a feeling is sometimes a sign of the incipient organization of a higher tendency, but in that case it invariably indicates that the higher tendency is not completely organized; thus the individual who experiences it may be described as superior, so far as complexity is concerned, to the man in whom the tendency does not as yet exist even in its rudimentary state and cannot produce any affective phenomenon; but he is inferior from the point of view of coherence and unity to the person in whom the tendency is sufficiently well organized to enter into activity and to terminate in action without disturbance or check, and consequently without an accompaniment of affective phenomena. An affective phenomena is the sign of a disturbance which may sometimes accompany an extension of systematization about to be effected in the organism, but it is always the sign of an imperfection and disorder of activity.

FEELING, INTELLIGENCE, AND WILL IN GENERAL PSYCHOLOGY

In many respects psychology has changed very little since it first began to receive attention. It still depends upon those few generalizations, somewhat old-fashioned and vague in their import, which served to found the science. We no longer describe feeling, intelligence and will as "faculties of the soul", but we still deal with them as groups of distinct and irreducible things. In spite of the endeavours of certain scientists, consciousness, the inmost sense, still retains a wide range of meaning against which strong objections may be raised. Its real nature, moreover, is insufficiently understood — even misunderstood ; nor is there agreement even as to its existence. It is interesting to note that the writers who would deny its reality or would assign to it scarcely any importance are precisely those who unwittingly endow it with an exaggerated importance and fail to recognize the dangers of their procedure. Although the problems of memory, habit, and instinct are sometimes treated from a fresh point of view and studied more closely and exhaustively than in former days, they seem to present much the same face as ever.

What is most lacking in the study of the mind, in the immense majority of cases, is a conception of mind itself. We have been told that physics does not deal with matter, nor physiology with life, and that in the same way there should be a "psychology without a soul". And perhaps this was right, if the object was to deprecate the search for substances, for things-in-themselves, for metaphysical entities, as our predecessors were pleased to conceive them some hundred years ago. But it would be wrong if it meant that we must abandon the endeavour to attain synthetic conceptions of the mind as a whole. I need not here concern myself very much with the doings of physics or biology in their own domains, but it seems to me that the physicists have made various interesting attempts to build up a synthetic idea of matter and the biologists of life. And if they had not made these attempts, they would have erred in neglecting an aspect of their sciences which has its practical interest, and which is of prime importance from a purely scientific point of view.

Thus psychology is marred by a two-fold deficiency of analysis and synthesis. Analysis is left incomplete, or, in the triumph of routine, is in many respects not even outlined. Synthesis is unproductive, or it is not attempted ; and the majority of psychologists do not even appear to regret its absence. Several syntheses have, indeed, been offered, but they have failed and been consigned to oblivion. Not long ago, Spencer proposed one which was imperfect and debatable, but interesting. It is forgotten, or very nearly so, without there being any occasion to combat it. The physiologists, and a few psychologists, desiring to refer psychical life to complicated reflexes, had at least pointed out a way of doing so. It is not altogether their fault if more progress has not been made in that direction. And as for the general views upon mind presented by Henri Bergson, there has been a tendency perhaps to utilize them in the interests of various creeds rather than to examine them for their own sake, and for the science of psychology as such.

We are doubtless very ready to believe that analysis, and especially observation, should precede the formulation of comprehensive views, and that psychology is still too young a science to be capable of expanding

into really fruitful synthetic conceptions.   And it would
be premature, to say the least of it, to claim that we
have already achieved any complete and final syntheses.
It is scarcely likely that man will ever attain to them.
But it is none the less true that observation, analysis,
and synthesis should be pursued simultaneously; that
synthesis would never be achieved if it were necessary
first to exhaust observation and analysis; that these
are frequently called forth or facilitated by it; moreover, that to have a conception of the circulation, for
example, it is not indispensable to have observed and
analysed all its phenomena down to the last detail;
and that we can perceive the causes, the general features
and the consequences of a war without being aware of
the doings of all the soldiers who have taken part in it.

I. *Intelligence, Feeling, and Will do not form distinct
groups of phenomena.*   When I endeavour to study the
real nature of psychical facts, I am struck by the lack of
accord between them and the assertions I find in books,
and by their apparent unwillingness to fit into the
divisions that have been prepared for them after a somewhat superficial examination, in accordance with conventions or traditions too strictly followed.   Certainly
these conventions and traditions have their use, but only
so long as they are modified, broadened, and adapted
at the same time, and, what is more, interpreted.
Sometimes they have been treated in this way with
tolerable success: for example, in the case of the relations between judgment, reasoning, and perception, and
the associations of memory, habit, and instinct.   Much
remains to be said upon these questions; and instinct,
for example, still has many mysteries.   But fuller
investigation and a thorough re-modelling are required
elsewhere; particularly with regard to certain general
characteristics of psychical facts, which serve to constitute the universally accepted groups, for the distinction
and relations between intelligence, feeling, and will.

In every psychological fact—if the words are properly understood, if, that is to say, they are used to denote what is really essential in the phenomena which they describe — we can discern feeling, intelligence, will, instinct, memory and invention. These words, then, should not, strictly speaking, be taken as designating groups of psychical facts : they denote certain characteristics which are encountered, in various degrees and under diverse forms, in all the groups and even in all the facts.

Let us take any example whatsoever ; say the solution of a simple problem in algebra. If this is not examined over-carefully, it may be grouped among the facts of an intellectual order ; and indeed intelligence is certainly involved. But there are also a number of affective elements present. From the outset it is conditioned by affective facts. Since we have made up our mind to apply ourselves to it, the problem interests us for some reason ; frequently, in some cases chiefly, for the sheer pleasure of working it out. Said Maupertuis, seated in his arm-chair, "I should like to solve a good problem which would not give me much trouble." In fact, in the actual process of pursuing a solution, we are more or less interested or even impassioned, and not always but sometimes 'moved'. There is pleasure in imagining combinations, in discovering the road that leads to the result, whilst pain, weariness and vexation lie in fruitless search, or in the sense that we are checked by some difficulty in the reasoning or the calculation. Here, then, intelligence and feeling are already engaged, but the solution of the problem also demands a constant activity of the will. Not only must we desire the end in view—the solution, and work to realize that desire, but also in some measure we must will each operation, each step forward, whether rightly directed or not, as well as occasional necessary backward steps and renewed endeavours ; if the problem is at all difficult, we are bound to reflect and deliberate, to make comparisons, to judge, determine, and to issue the 'fiat' with which philosophers of will are concerned. And all this hangs together; it forms a whole. The exercise of the intelligence cannot be separated from that of feeling or of will: they can only be separated, that is to say, by an abstraction which isolates the sundry aspects of a single fact, the different sides of the same geometrical figure. Our ideas summon up or *will* other ideas; they are accompanied by a special pleasure or annoyance which adheres to them, so to speak, and can only be disengaged from them by artificial means.

It must be added that a part of the facts produced, a part even of their intellectual side, more or less escapes our knowledge, and that we do not think of observing this, and have only a kind of abstract feeling of it. (Note the meaning attached to the term 'a feeling'— *sentiment*—in which intelligence and sensibility are equally involved, and also, probably, will.) [1] Moreover, in the solution of a problem memory, habit, and routine play a relatively large part, though this may consist merely in the recognition and handling of letters, numbers and formulæ, while the function of invention is relatively limited.

Thus feeling, intelligence, will, instinct, habit, memory, invention, reasoning, and judgment are united and mingled, even in a relatively simple matter which may at first appear to be no more than a minor process of pure intelligence. Observation and analysis can undoubtedly disentangle them; but in reality they are firmly united and, in certain respects, inseparable. This, I hope, will appear still more clearly at a later stage.

Conversely, let us take what everyone admits to be a feeling and our observations will be analogous. But we are immediately struck by the want of precision in

---

[1] *Sensibilité* has been translated, as occasion demanded, by either 'sensibility' or 'feeling'; while *sentiment* (*cf.* p. 65, note) is usually equivalent to 'a feeling'.—*Translator's note.*

psychological language and in the ideas that it represents. No one will regard love as a fact of an intellectual order : if there be any 'feeling' where title is not in dispute it is certainly to be found here. But a feeling of love, taken in its complexity, has many phases which differ considerably in nature and value. It springs up and generally develops in a somewhat irregular manner, reaches its apogee (a state which varies greatly, according to the circumstances), then abates gradually, or suddenly, and takes on a new form, although it may still be given the old name ; sometimes it returns, flames up again, and dies down. Moreover, even while it endures and flourishes, it does not constantly occupy the mind ; sometimes it is especially intense, and at other times a little dulled ; it invades the spirit and then retires, as does the tide from the shore. It organizes a countless multitude of varied phenomena, which are really an integral part of it : ideas, dreams, emotions, wishes, actions, suppositions and perceptions, images and judgments, reasonings and recollections. Habit, memory, routine, instinct, and also invention, are continually in evidence during the process. All this is systematized around a kind of governing instinct, the sexual tendency, more or less specialized for a time at any rate, and directed towards a single being. But it is this whole assemblage of diverse experiences that constitutes a passion, a feeling, and if we try to separate them from the feeling, it no longer exists. What would love be without some knowledge of the person loved, without imaginative schemes, projects, dreams—in other words, without intellectual experiences? It would not exist either as love or as feeling, and would be reduced, or would tend to be reduced, to a mere blind impulse, headlong and indiscriminate : in short, it would be suppressed. But then, again, what would it be without the volitions which conduce either to its gratification, or to its more or less indirect development or diminution? Intelligence and will seem to be as essential to feeling as feeling and will are to intelligence. Even a fairly summary observation and analysis prove them to be inseparable.

If, now, instead of taking a complex feeling with an elaborate history, we examine an element of this feeling, still with a distinctly affective character, we get a similar result. The emotion experienced at the sight of a person we love, for example, condenses or develops many ideas, and it is, in itself, an element of volition. It would not be the thing it is without the memories which it to some extent awakens, without a recognition of the person, and consequently without an intelligent elaboration of the perception.

We should obtain similar results from studying the development of a feeling of envy, or of a sudden impression of fear. Furthermore, a 'feeling' is accompanied, obviously enough, by some consciousness that is inherent in it, a consciousness that may be confused or distinct, erroneous or veracious. But consciousness is a kind of knowledge, and knowledge is pre-eminently an intellectual experience. From this angle we again arrive at the conclusion that some intellectual process is essential to a feeling which is not reduced to an absolutely unconscious tendency.

All this would seem to indicate that it is impossible in practice to separate the concrete facts of intelligence, feeling, and will, and to suggest that they are different faces of a single fact, or merely what one sees when regarding it in different ways. Perhaps, too, it will already be suspected that the three traditional faculties do not express the essential functioning of the mind, but different modes or qualities of something that is deeper and more substantial.

II. *Feeling and Consciousness.* To resume our analysis. It is certainly true that we do not take exact account of the feelings which we experience nor of all that goes

with them.   And it is easy enough for us to contrast
enlightened intelligence with blind passion.   But we
fail to realize that in doing this we are not so much
contrasting feeling with intelligence as one form of
intelligence with another form of intelligence, and one
form of feeling with another form of feeling.   There
is no such thing as lucid intelligence without affective
impressions, and it may even be inspired by passion
and take a keen pleasure in exercising and developing
itself.   Blind passion may accompany or call forth
false ideas, but it never occurs without ideas, images,
dreams, and even opinions and arguments.   In a
sense we may say that passion is always, in itself and
in certain respects, knowledge (or error) and at the
same time that it is no less essentially volition.   This
will be more apparent later on.

Again, it is certainly possible to be afraid without
quite realizing it, and erotic emotion is not always
distinctly accepted for what it is.   Not only may the
new tendency which calls it forth continue to be misunderstood, but even the attraction may not be clearly
realized.

In this case, however, the feeling is not quite what
it would be if it were accurately appraised.   A feeling
consciously understood is always to some extent transformed.   When it is better known, it is no longer
experienced in entirely the same way, but is weakened
or enriched by certain elements, and new reactions
take place within it : it calls forth fresh associations
and dissociations, and finds relationships and opposi-
tions among other elements, which more or less transform
it.   The intellectual experience is not foreign to the
affective fact, but is superadded to it as a kind of
epiphenomenon.   Both are closely united, and what
we term a fact of feeling, an affective fact, or an intellectual fact, is like a chemical combination in which
all the elements are essential.

The affective fact could not dispense with intellectual

elements, even though these be not recognized. They are, indeed, never completely known or perfectly comprehended. We cannot here enter into the problem of the 'unconscious'; but it may be remarked that a great part of our psychical life, and also a relatively important part of each phenomenon, remains unknown to us. But when a conscious fact is produced, it is an essential character of this fact, without which it would not be conscious, that, with a greater or lesser degree of clarity and completeness, it is perceived, recognized and taken up by an intellectual operation, an internal perception, the mechanism of which—as I have often had occasion to note—is similar in essentials to that of external perception.

It may be argued, perhaps, that the affective fact is in itself unconscious. If anyone actually holds that view he is at liberty to defend it. We can only say that the same can be said of the intellectual fact, and we then approach the conception which makes intellectual, affective, and volitional facts, as they are generally understood, relatively clear and well-differentiated accompaniments of tendency, always largely unconscious. If feeling be regarded as conscious, it is unquestionable that it involves in some measure an intellectual process.

III. *Inter-relationships of Intelligence and Feeling.* The psychologist constantly has to establish affinities, resemblances, and identities, which have been insufficiently considered, between intellectual and affective facts. It is significant that Ribot, who on several occasions insisted upon the differences and contrasts between feeling and intelligence, was nevertheless constrained to deal with topics such as affective memory, affective imagination, and even the logic of feelings, upon which he wrote one of his best books. Affective and intellectual facts are, indeed, not only so inseparable as to be actually confused in certain respects, but also they are subject to the same general psychological laws. They are cast in the same moulds of life, and evince similar qualities—so similar that each order exhibits qualities which appear to be the special characteristics of the other. This is an additional reason for suspecting that a radical distinction cannot be drawn between them in the way which is commonly adopted. We find in them resemblances and even particularly arresting identities, which should put us in the way of a general conception of psychological facts.

Some of them, though not in the first rank of importance, are nevertheless interesting. Thus we hear much talk of acuteness of intelligence as well as of acuteness of feeling, or of the refinement, bluntness, subtlety, clumsiness, rapidity, or slowness of these faculties.

But the special characteristic which shows the primary identity, in certain respects, of facts belonging to different classes, is that we constantly recognize in feelings qualities which indicate intelligence, and still more perhaps, in ideas, characters belonging to the order of sensibility.

We all know what is meant by 'blind passions', 'wise discretion', 'reasonable desires', 'insane ambitions', 'enlightened virtues'. On the other hand, we are acquainted also with 'sensitive' intellects; 'passionate', 'fiery', 'hasty', 'calm' minds; 'cool' and 'ardent' thought.

This is not simply a question of metaphors or of adjectives qualifying the whole of a personality exhibiting the feeling or idea to which qualities of another order are imputed by a figure of speech. A sensitive intellect is not necessarily the intellect of a personality in whom other forms of sensibility are very keen. Indeed, there are certain people whose intelligence is more 'sensitive' than their affectionate, domestic, or patriotic tendencies. Fontenelle seems to have been one of these, and possibly, with certain reservations, Goethe. "You have a brain instead of a heart", was once said to a representative of the same type; and that expresses the matter, roughly, perhaps, but plainly.

A sensitive intelligence is one which a very slight stimulus suffices to set in action, and which reacts in various ways to very small differences in the stimulus. Intelligence has ended by producing a tendency, just as any other faculty can do, which manifests itself in man and in certain men especially;[1] and, as a whole, it is no more distinct from sensibility than any other tendency —love of one's family, for example, patriotism, or sexual desire. It has its own sensibility, and in a way it may be regarded as a form of sensibility (just as, from another point of view, we might recognize in sensibility a form of intelligence, and, in both, forms of will). Its sensibility is distinct and variable according to the individual and also, for the same individual, according to circumstances. Some minds are very sensitive to literature and scarcely sensitive at all to mathematics. Pascal, though he possessed an admirable combination of the geometrical mind and the cultured mind, was obliged to enlist the assistance of friends to develop his intellectual sensibility in the latter respect, and this process of education was swiftly accomplished. Each intellect has its own emotional power, its desires, and its tastes. We may be fascinated by an idea no less than by a picture or a woman. There are intellects which are continually excited, impassioned and agitated (Proudhon, Lamennais); others that are interested in ideas and things somewhat as the gourmet appreciates an exquisite dish, or the amateur a beautiful piece of china (Sainte-Beuve, for instance, or Faguet, who was a great amateur of ideas); and there are others of dull sensibility, who

---

[1] See, on this subject, *Les types intellectuels, esprits logiques et esprits faux*, in which I have studied the differentiation and organization of the intellectual tendency among the other tendencies.

remain indifferent and interested in very little, who live
in a cold and torpid fashion, sensitive only to organic
desire or the need for love or wealth. But once these
people are stirred to activity, they also display an
individual and frequently characteristic sensibility.

Intellectual emotion is the mark of one order of mind,
and it distinguishes the 'intellectuals'. Among them
especially we may find genuine 'characters' of the intelligence, analogous to the complete human characters
—those which determine personality. Illustrations of
this general fact will occur to everyone. Michelet had an
impassioned, bold and adventurous intellect, Voltaire's
was very sensitive, quick and irascible, John Stuart
Mill's calm and reflective.

In the same way, there are blind feelings and clear-
sighted feelings. There are stupid passions which
nothing can enlighten, and which not only injure the
entire personality but also defeat their own ends.
Others, more rare, are circumspect, disciplined, and
able to rectify themselves in case of need, but they
tend to be naturally intelligent, reason well after a
fashion, and display a steady and consistent logical
sequence.

The person in whom these different feelings exist
does not always possess their qualities and their defects
in any precise sense. There are plenty of examples of
a blind love in a mind generally clear. And, on the
other hand, in certain persons of mediocre intelligence,
some desires are clever and prudent, and find a way of
adapting themselves to circumstances, of modifying or
accommodating them to suit their purposes.

Just as there are true ideas and false ideas, so it may
be said that there are also true feelings and false
feelings. I do not intend this in a moral sense; I
mean rather that some feelings have a true sort of
understanding and others a false. The former have a
sense of reality and adapt themselves to it, whereas the
latter go contrary to their own ends, and act incon-

sistently. Persons who possess the first, for example, know instinctively how to choose their friends, and, even without reflection, do not bestow their confidence and esteem, or even their love, in a misguided way. Others have incoherent feelings, out of harmony with reality and with themselves, and are incapable of perceiving or correcting their mistakes.

Thus it may be said with some degree of accuracy that every intelligence, every idea even, has its sensibility, its own peculiar character; whilst every feeling has its own intelligence, lucidity, blindness, and folly.

IV. *The Volitional aspect.* Intelligence and feeling have likewise their 'will'; and will, apart from feeling and intelligence, obviously does not exist. An activity without ideas or emotions would be at best a reflex activity. An activity without any sort of discernment or sensibility would be an incomprehensible freak, if, indeed, it could be anything at all.

That feeling has, if not its 'will' in the strict sense, at least its predetermined aim, its tendency, and its direction, is clear even from casual observation. It is most abundantly evident that the passions 'will' to be satisfied, that avarice 'wills' riches, that ambition 'wills' power, glory, and grandeur, that love 'wills' love. Although the influence of other special wills and of antagonistic desires may be an obstacle in their path, and although the superior will of the organized mind may precipitate, arrest, or suspend manifestation, that in no way prevents particular tendencies from existing by themselves as decided and sharply-defined wills, which seek expression in appropriate actions if nothing counteracts them.

We may go further. The formation of a feeling closely resembles the beginning of a volition. Without doubt, our feelings usually develop in an almost unconscious way; but our actions, for the most part, are also performed without the intervention of any conscious and deliberate act of volition. This only appears after a certain interval, after a certain amount of consideration and a more or less facile calculation. We encounter all these factors again in the formation of certain feelings, which are hesitant at first, so that it is not easy to say what definite form they will take. Friendship, confidence, love, piety, do not always appear like a bolt from the blue; the feeling is outlined and developed, it recedes or it feels its way, until at a given moment, under the influence of external circumstances, of varied reflections, ideas, and impressions, crystallization takes place, and it is established in a more or less durable fashion : the confidence, friendship or love exists and is affirmed ; we may say, in a sense, that it is 'willed'. Its birth is similar to the formation of a volition which establishes a mental attitude. In both cases, a decision is taken, the consequences of which will be felt later.

But if feelings 'will' and 'are willed' it is the same with intelligence and ideas. Ideas have tendencies, like feelings : they seek and summon each other ; a series of ideas inevitably calls up one idea but absolutely repels others. We can sum up their action by saying that the premises of a syllogism will the conclusion. Systematic association is the law of healthy intelligence, as of all healthy psychical activity ; this will of ideas which creates other ideas, annexes them to itself, and places them in groups, is perpetually at work, and in certain respects it characterizes the whole of intellectual activity.

Ideas do not will ideas only : they also will actions and feelings. If the idea is sensibility, it is also action, and all possible kinds of action. It is a grave error to deny it this characteristic. The idea of an action is already a tendency to action. One of the great merits of Fouillée was to remind us of this motor, practical, and positive aspect of ideas, and to establish and illustrate it.

Here again, undoubtedly, obstacles frequently intervene and veil the nature and working of the elements. An idea is a tendency ; other tendencies, ideas, feelings, or the superior will of the personality, may impede its flight, or prevent its complete realization. The tendency is none the less real. If checked, it is interpreted in the intellectual domain by the reflections, thoughts, and images which accumulate so frequently in the mind of man under the influence of desires or apprehensions, acquired beliefs, or predominant ideas ; for example— by the reduction of a practical idea to ineffectual projects, dreams, and ' castles in the air '.

At the very moment it wills, the idea ' is willed '. Intellectual activity often assumes an automatic, half unconscious form, like affective and indeed all human activity ; and it also allows of volitions, entirely similar to and essentially identical with the volitions of practical activity. Most of our ideas are constituted without any attention, or at least if there is any attention paid to the idea itself there is none for the process by which it is formed ; just as the majority even of our conscious actions are decided upon without our noticing, or if we do notice the decisions made, we know nothing of their genesis. But when we have to perform a difficult, unusual or debatable action, or to grasp an important but also debatable and as yet unproven theory, or to solve a weighty problem, then it is that we see intellectual volition arising, like practical or moral volition. Cohesion of ideas is not obtained at the outset. We will set aside the case where belief is involved, since it is too complex and may possibly bring factors other than ideas into operation. But where there is a problem, ideas seek and invoke other ideas, they hazard incomplete and imperfect solutions, provisional systems which will disappear or prepare the way for better systems. This sort of deliberation may last for a long time, and then, in fortunate cases, the desired idea at length comes to complete, reorganize, and establish the system. Everything is in order, the crystallization is effected, the positive volition is achieved. Perhaps its influence will long re-echo in the mind and promote fresh adjustments, new forms of thought. And each one of the systems thus fashioned abruptly or gradually, consciously or by a kind of instinctive genius, is yet willed, in the sense that it tends, of its own accord, to persist indefinitely—a tendency which is, however, also opposed and occasionally checked, as in the case of the will to act, by latent or open discord of the elements, and by appeals from other quarters.

If then there is action everywhere in the mind and, in a sense, voluntary action, if everywhere there is intelligence and everywhere sensibility, clearly the old and still respected division of psychical facts into three groups, or their reference to three or four faculties, must be abandoned, modified, or explained.

V. *Mental operations.* We will endeavour in due course to examine the conclusions which follow from this. But first, it is not without interest to raise certain other psychological questions. If instead of devoting ourselves to the nature of the phenomena, we study them in their relations and take into consideration the workings of the mind, our conclusions will agree with those we have just discovered.

Whatever mental operation we are considering and whatever be its outcome, it seems clear that we can find its precise equivalents in all the orders of psychical facts. And, if we are working on general lines, we are also able to recognize them in each of the phenomena grouped in these different orders.

For example, we are aware that there is reasoning in all mental processes, and from this point of view psychologists have often successfully reconciled phenomena which were considered to be very different. With regard to perception, there remains scarcely any doubt, and here we need only refer to the psychological system of Wundt and to Binet's well-known study. There is reasoning also in feelings and affections, inasmuch as it has been possible to write a volume on the logic of feelings, which, valuable though it is, has not by any means exhausted the subject. An emotion is the conclusion of a kind of special syllogism, in which a tendency, passion, or feeling is the major, the minor being a given circumstance, an internal or external event,[1] the appearance of a person, the sight of an object, the coming of an unforeseen idea, or the disturbance due to another feeling.

There is no need to demonstrate the fact that logic exists in our will and in our actions. An action, voluntary or instinctive, is the conclusion necessitated by the relations established between the tendencies, feelings, desires, and ideas, between the ego and the circumstances in which its activity has to be exercised. I am hungry, and dinner is served ; it is logical for me to go to the table. Harpagon is miserly : he sees two candles burning ; it is logical for him to blow one of

---

[1] Indeed, from this point of view, everything may appear as the conclusion of a syllogism, of which the major is a fact, especially an antecedent general fact, and the minor a new circumstance or a new conjunction of circumstances. Major : a small balloon which I hold in my hand is filled with a gas lighter than air : minor, I open my fingers : conclusion, the balloon escapes. The order of the facts is similar to the order of ideas in reasoning ; that is to say, when the observation is good and the reasoning accurate, the one precisely corresponds to the other. I do not believe that no inference can be drawn from this, but I abstain here from philosophical deductions.

I would only remark that all determinism thus assumes a logical form, in which the antecedents represent the major, the final alteration the minor, and what results from it is necessarily the conclusion. A series of indeterminate phenomena would represent something like a reasoning process, incoherent in character, which would be logical only by a prodigious series of chances ; and even then, the indeterminate series, however logical, could not be distinguished from an absolutely determined series. Thus if in roulette we were to obtain by chance the first fifteen figures of the number π, the result would be in no way distinguishable from a series conditioned by the will of a mathematician to give the number π as far as the sixteenth figure. The two cases are not identical, since the second shows the absence of a determining condition, and the first the absence of all determination : but they are comparable, and the first is a sort of limiting case of the second.

L

them out. Thus, each of our actions may be referred to
the conclusion of a sort of syllogism, which is more or
less complex and also more or less conscious. Neither
the most instinctive nor the most 'free' of our actions
escape this view; and though it is perfectly justifiable
to regard them from another standpoint, the new point
of view ought not to displace the first, but should
merely be combined with it and with others.

Moreover, the premises of the active syllogism are
extremely complex; but the premises of intellectual
reasoning are not always so simple as those which
logicians find it convenient to give us. Thanks to this
and certain other observations, we may admit that there
is also reasoning in intelligence; for it is very certain
that the syllogism, as it appears in treatises on logic, is
never employed in its explicit and theoretical form.
This, however, is not our problem here, and the
reasoning which we are considering is an implicit
reasoning, or rather a combination of psychical facts,
which may be cast into the mould of the syllogism, but
which generally originates and develops in complete
disregard of it. And it is often rather amusing to
see the clumsy form into which an argument is put by
persons with insufficient training. Obviously, if the
word were given too narrow a sense we should no longer
discover reasoning in action, in feeling, or even in
perception, and in the end we might no longer find it
in living reality except in very rare circumstances—
perhaps not at all.

We have not yet had occasion to consider those
complex cases in which feelings and ideas are more
obviously blended—for example, the case of a conversion, a change of belief, in which the whole
personality is involved. Although these are very
significant, I have preferred to approach the question
by examples in which the interpretation, though perhaps
less easy, was for that very reason more convincing
and significant. On the famous night when Jouffroy

renounced his beliefs, which prevailed—his intellect, his love of truth, or his will? Without doubt all three were inextricably mingled ; which leads us again to suspect that the same fact is at once a manifestation of sensibility, an application of the intelligence, and an act of the will, according as it is regarded from one side or the other and in relation to some other particular phenomenon—somewhat as a man may be both the father of a family and at the same time a member of the town council.

VI. *Memory, Invention, Instinct, and Imagination.* Furthermore, we find memory everywhere. There is not one of our feelings, our ideas, or our volitions, which fails to reproduce something of the past. We discover recollections in the most original invention, routine and instinct in the most premeditated action of the will. And this is why it is necessary to come to an understanding as to the meaning of the term ' organized memory' which is sometimes used. There is undoubtedly a certain organization in the facts of memory—to some extent in all of them, but more especially in some. But memory is one thing, organization another, and they are constantly combined though always distinguishable. They are like intelligence and sensibility —different relations existing in a single complex fact, and connecting it with others while linking up its elements. Memory implies organization, but by itself it is not organization, it is persistence. Persistence, however, is a condition of mental organization, which in its turn is something quite other than persistence. On the one hand, organization is necessary to memory and is found even in what Dugas calls ' brute' memory. On the other hand, if memory is necessary to organization, it often also contradicts it ; that is to say, a higher organization is frequently hindered or confused by the persistence of elementary organizations.

If, moreover, we consider in a somewhat haphazard fashion facts such as invention, imagination, instinct, imitation, caprice, which we are often disposed to refer to a single class of phenomena, we find that they adjust themselves to all the categories, and that they also not infrequently combine among themselves, even when they appear to be opposed and contradictory. There is no invention without imitation and routine, no imitation or routine that does not embody a few infinitesimal particles of invention, no volition that is not based upon instincts.

But above all, our principal concern here is our belief that every operation admits at the same time of feeling, intelligence, and will. Feelings are invented, like ideas, and actions, like feelings. Strictly speaking, will is a sort of practical invention. There are persons in whose feelings routine is very powerful, and who offer special proof of affective imitation, while others create tastes and affections for themselves, and experience them in an original and personal manner. One may experience a commonplace love or a love rare and peculiar, a vulgar ambition or an ambition which is strange and little known, and therefore little understood. This refers not only to the object of the feeling and the purpose towards which it draws a man, but also to its constituent elements, to qualities which are sometimes difficult to define (for example, a mixture of charm, vigour, and tenacity)—to its movement and rhythm.

Instinct is related rather to practical activity. But it will readily be admitted that it exists also in affective life, and that most of our feelings are in a large measure instinctive. And it is beyond question that there are also intellectual instincts : we can constantly witness their activity in ourselves and others. Our tendencies towards analysis, observation, and synthesis are very clearly defined as instincts. It is the same with certain methods of reasoning peculiar to different men or different groups, and also with our special preferences and aptitudes for observing or employing ideas or abstract images, concrete images of a special kind, certain words, etc.

Imagination is also omnipresent. Although, understanding the word in its ordinary sense, we may consider it as a tendency to create, revive, or combine images which very often have no immediate practical utility and stand somewhat apart from real life, we nevertheless know perfectly well that the images may represent feelings, decisions, and volitions, as well as all sorts of facts, and that they are therefore not merely ideas and intellectual figures, but also outlines, more or less lifelike and incisive, of feelings and actions. Observations of this kind could be multiplied indefinitely.

THE NATURE OF FEELING, INTELLIGENCE, AND WILL

I. *Feeling*

IT may seem that the chief result of our analysis has been to mingle and confuse facts which were supposed to be comparatively clear. It will now be our task to build up a new and, if possible, more real and enduring order.

If feeling, intelligence, and will are not groups of distinct facts, what are they? They might be mere phantoms. But that is very improbable, and we cannot but think that a characterization so generally accepted must correspond to some solid reality. But as we have suggested, they may also be abstract elements of facts, different relations existing between the elements of those facts, or between the elements or the facts themselves and other facts, or the elements of other facts.

If we investigate the most general and essential qualities of those facts to which the term feeling or sensibility is usually applied, we find a disposition to react under the influence of a stimulus from within or without. Sensibility measures in some degree the facility, vivacity, and intensity of this reaction. It is to be noted that the reaction, in connection with the human mind, may remain internal, at least in appearance, and not be transferred to the exterior by any readily appreciable phenomenon. Sensitiveness to reproaches, for example, may be made manifest in some persons by a stamping of the feet, or by tears and cries, and in others by prolonged and silent reflection or secret remorse. The latter type is not necessarily the less sensitive.

It seems to me that this definition covers all the

features customarily assigned to sensibility, or at any
rate all their essential qualities, while at the same time
it distinguishes sensibility from other properties of
psychical phenomena, and allows us to understand
their relations. It must not be supposed, however,
that our definition is perfect; it must be interpreted,
completed, and adapted, possibly to the extent of intro-
ducing some trifling contradiction, which we must
endeavour to reduce to insignificance or at any rate to
recognize in order to avoid its perils.

There can be no doubt that what is generally termed
sensibility is just this possibility of reaction which I
have indicated. A 'sensitive' man is one who reacts
to the least stimulus, by emotions and movements : and
doubtless there are many ways of being sensitive. The
selfish or heedless sensibility of some persons may be
contrasted with the kindly sensibility of others ; the
former might be called impressionable. But we certainly
observe a general character corresponding to the general
term.

Proceeding to details, sensibility viewed as the
activity of the perceptive apparatus, for example, is
included in our group. This is obviously a question of
reaction (internal, and translated also into various
movements) to a stimulus from without (external perception) or from within (internal perception, inner sense,
consciousness)—a reaction of the organism and of the
mind. As regards the relation of sensation and perception
to intelligence and sensibility, I would only remark that
they appertain to sensibility in so far as they disclose a
possibility of reaction on the part of some being, and
to intelligence in so far as they are knowledge, and
introduce into the mind a representation (exact or otherwise, symbolic or otherwise) of some internal or external
reality. But we shall examine this last point more
carefully when we are dealing with intelligence.

Sensibility, as the faculty of experiencing pleasure
and pain, still exhibits a reaction. We describe its

characteristics when we speak of sensibility as being, on the one hand, more keen or delicate, or on the other, coarser or duller, in proportion as the reaction is more or less prompt, exact, or extensive; or again in proportion as the stimulus is quick or slow to call forth pleasure and pain, no matter whether it be very slight or whether in order not to be ineffective it has to be much stronger; or, finally, in proportion as the pleasure and pain are more or less keen and intense.

Attempts have been made to reduce sensibility to this potentiality for pleasure and pain.[1] This would restrict its compass to a remarkable degree, but it does not, however, misrepresent the nature of pain and pleasure. They are most essentially a response of the mind to a group of circumstances. Like sensibility, they may be described as the power to experience various emotions, inclinations, and passions. The most important thing in this connection is the internal reaction of the mind to a given situation, the readiness with which the mind is modified or modifies some of its elements in response to some stimulus, apart from the active and co-ordinated reaction which may follow, and which is dependent upon the will. We shall consider the will later on, but even at this stage it is easy to understand that an individual may have much sensibility and little will. That is to say, his mind reacts to stimuli with emotions, imaginative combinations, vivid impressions, and perhaps with tears, cries, and unco-ordinated movements, but he is scarcely able to systematize his mental states into a positive volition and act so as to adapt himself to the stimuli or to adapt them to his desires. But it is evident that sensibility always involves a certain mental activity, which is one of the forms of will in its widest sense.

Hence we say that sensibility is keener or greater according to the ease with which the passions are aroused in a given individual; and that it is fuller and

[1] Cf. Léon Dumont, *Théorie scientifique de la sensibilité*.

deeper according to the strength, variety, intensity, and permanence of the passions, inclinations, and tastes : more delicate and subtle according as the emotions and impressions are more finely shaded, more diverse, and associated with slighter stimuli, whose smallest changes and details they interpret.   A man has a sensitive taste, for example, if he can detect the difference between the same wine of a different vintage ; he possesses sensitive literary feeling if he appreciates authors who are given to subtlety of expression, and if he is aware of their variable and intricate charm.   In all this we are concerned simply with different expressions of the same phenomenon.

We shall now have no difficulty in recognizing sensibility in groups of facts which on other accounts seemed to exclude it.   Our definition is applicable not only to all those which have invariably been regarded as dependent on it, but it also explains the presence of sensibility in groups from which it has been excluded and to which it has been opposed.

Take, for example, intellectual facts.   It may appear singular to make perception depend upon sensibility, and imagination upon intelligence ; but that is only because the external stimulus is more immediate and obvious in perception.   Intelligence has its sensibility none the less, and in certain respects we might say that it is a feeling.   Every idea, every image, every argument, is also in one aspect a response of the mind to a challenge from the world, the organism or the mind itself, and is therefore from this point of view a fact of sensibility, as much as perception or emotion.   Moreover, we shall not be surprised to find that intelligences and even ideas, systems of notions, and images can be relatively sensitive and swiftly awakened, or on the contrary relatively slow, torpid, or idle.   Voltaire belonged to a type of quick intellectual sensibility, and we have all met with intellects of dull sensibility, difficult to move and indifferent to a great many stimuli. The sensitiveness of the intellect, like that of the feelings, will seem the more active, according as ideas spring up more speedily and easily; the more profound or broad, according as the stimulus produces a more enduring reaction and extends to a wider or remoter sphere of thought; the more subtle, according as stimuli which differ only slightly are provocative of distinct ideas. And it is not without interest to recall that the "faculty of experiencing pleasure and pain" belongs also to the intellect, and may, with reservations, afford an approximate measure of its sensibility. But not only are there intellectual pleasures and pains: the intellect likewise possesses its tastes, inclinations and passions. It is scarcely necessary to recall the different vocations of different minds, the passion for poetry and mathematics, the taste for art, the inveterate tendency towards observation or analysis, or to cite in evidence the great intellectuals[1] of all time. It would thus appear somewhat curious that cold and lucid intelligence (sometimes it is neither the one nor the other) should have been so persistently contrasted with blind feeling, did we not know how easy and usual it is to neglect obvious facts and to uphold a theory that ignores them. Everyone was certainly aware that intelligence was something sensitive, and that sensibility might have its clarity of vision, but recognition of this fact was studiously avoided lest it should disturb a convention.

The sensibility of the will is no less real, though it has perhaps received even less attention than the sensibility of the intelligence, for a reason which will appear more plainly later on; and we shall find this new field no less rich in material. Some wills can

---

[1] Here I give this word its correct meaning. It denotes persons in whom the exercise of the intelligence is the dominant tendency and governs at least the greater part of their lives. It may happen that the intellectual is not intelligent. I have also known people who were devoted to sport, but proved very unskilful at it.

be more readily stimulated than others ; some are slow and inactive, others refined or coarse, tender or brutish, hasty or sluggish. The act of volition, the decision, is arrived at in very different ways, according to circumstances, no doubt, but also according to the nature of the mind in question. This internal reaction in the presence of a stimulus, in response to a concurrence of external and internal circumstances, also shows how sensibility varies from one mind to another. In some a decision is reached by a sort of swift and sudden crystallization, in others it admits of much groping and wavering. In some it will be subtly differentiated and particularized, in others it will be rough and ready, invariable in very different cases, occasionally even though the intellect may perceive the differences, and fairly sharp and varied affective impressions may arise in reference to them. It appears indeed that in certain persons the will has not the same sensibility as the intelligence and feelings, that it is more awkward and undiscriminating. Thus, certain qualities and certain defects are entirely peculiar to the sensibility of the will : they may even be said to characterize the activity which is directed towards the external or internal world for the purpose of transforming it and stamping it with a personal imprint, the activity, that is to say, which constitutes conduct. One may think vigorously, feel strongly, and act amiss. The volitional and active synthesis does not in these cases display the same sensibility as the syntheses of ideas and impressions.

Volitional sensitivity may also vary with the different tendencies of the same individual. Certain persons make up their minds quickly and successfully in particular kinds of activity, while in others they are listless, slow of will, and unsuccessful. Presently, moreover, we shall again encounter a truth of which we have already had a glimpse, namely, that the form of activity which determines conduct is not the only one in which volition manifests itself, and that there is also a kind of intellectual will, as well as a kind of affective will.

Since sensibility is essentially a response of the mind to a given set of circumstances, expressing at once the nature of the circumstances and that of the subject, it is obvious that it is omnipresent. This explains why certain authors have believed that they had discovered in sensibility the one essential and fundamental phenomenon from which all others are derived, and of which all others are only manifestations. Other writers, for similar reasons, have wished to attribute the same pre-eminence to the intellect—a view which is little in favour at present: or, again, to the will, a view which special circumstances once favoured and which would to-day, I believe, receive more support. We will confine ourselves to presenting sensibility as an essential element of every psychical fact. Where psychology has gone wrong has been in noticing this character for the most part in facts where there was no other to attract attention. It is facts of this sort which have tended to be referred to a special faculty or placed in a separate category.

We must revert for a while to the relations of sensibility and will, which are subtle and rather difficult to specify. Sensibility is the condition of will, and it is doubtless also one of its elements, just as it is a condition and an element of intelligence. We defined it by the reaction of the mind. But this reaction, without ever being absolutely passive, as it is too commonly represented—how could a reaction be entirely passive?—does not always present the characters and the high degree of systematization of voluntary action. Sensibility denotes that the mind may be stirred into activity after stimulation, and it signalizes the effect which that stimulation produces in it, an effect which is in itself a reaction manifesting the peculiar nature of the mind. Will is the co-ordinated reaction of the mind to deal with a situation by utilizing the impression left by the stimulus ; and, of course, the boundaries between sensibility and will are not always definite. Indeed, every fact of sensibility might be regarded as a fact of will, because it is a systematized response of the mind and the organism ; and it might be said that perception is the will of the apparatus that produces it. We might likewise consider every fact of will as a fact of sensibility —of cerebral and internal sensibility : for volition is also the response which external stimuli call forth from the organism and the mind. This is primarily a difference in point of view, but sometimes it is advantageous to regard one set of facts from a particular angle and another from a different one. If we are bent on finding a real difference, it will perforce be very abstract. We might say, for example, that sensibility is chiefly the mind's potentiality for being influenced by any external circumstance, organic or psychical ; and that will, on the other hand, is the mind's potentiality for influencing external events, organic or psychical. But the condition of mind which is influenced by another fact is likewise a systematized reaction that can in its turn influence other phenomena, transform them or produce them. And if the one reason would range it with sensibility, the other would make it a sort of volition. We shall then classify it according as one or other character predominates or impresses us more forcibly, or also according to convenience, remembering that if necessary it can be transferred.

Our perception of the relations of sensibility and will is somewhat confused, so much so that facts of activity, even the most characteristic phenomena of will are frequently interpreted in terms of sensibility, indicating, if not that they belong to sensibility, at least that they are the signs of sensibility. It is very common to see the sensibility of a person judged by his voluntary actions, and by his automatic or reflex activity. And, of course, except where we ourselves are concerned—in which case we may still be mistaken in various ways—this is the only means by which we can appraise the sensibility of a person. We can scarcely believe that sensibility is very keen when it does not reveal itself by any action or external sign (reflex movements, facial contraction, cries, various gestures, confidences, etc.). Often, moreover, this is a perfectly legitimate way of judging, and we can quite fairly impute lack of sensibility in certain respects to people who remain absolutely calm in certain circumstances. It may, however, lead to error. Some persons feel deeply, yet are incapable of action, and only betray their sensations by imperceptible or at least unperceived signs. The syntheses which are readily formed in them are not those which lead to actions, but are chiefly syntheses of ideas and impressions which may be very abundant; and their very richness and differentiation, causing the mind to be more satisfied by them, may render them more powerless, so that they become a source of gratification and a sort of end in themselves. It is then a form of æsthetic sensibility which is developed.

In the case of minds which are masters of themselves, prudent, circumspect minds, which calculate far in advance, immediate active manifestations are repressed and sensibility appears to be completely lacking, but, after a long delay, the concealed and powerful ideas and feelings will bring about the expedient voluntary action — revenge, for instance, carefully prepared in all its detail by long-standing malice. But it is also true that a certain want of sensibility, a genuine indifference, is not without its uses in the constitution of a strong, steady, and sufficiently healthy will. For the attainment of some important and remote object, it is good to be endowed naturally with a supreme indifference to the innumerable trifling incidents which might tend to divert us from it. And if nature has not furnished us with this indifference, we must know how to acquire it or to stimulate it—which is, besides, a means of acquiring it. We find illustrations of these points in pathological or semi-pathological cases where the will is powerless, though the sensibility remains keen. The conclusive synthesis does not succeed in establishing itself; it is replaced by a great number of imaginative and affective syntheses which, in themselves, may be considered as so many minor special volitions, but which, regarded as a whole, clearly indicate the superiority of sensibility over practical activity and the impotence of the will.

In concluding this section it may be noticed that this conception of sensibility is also applicable to those cases where the term sensibility is bestowed on phenomena of the inorganic world. If we say that salts of silver are 'sensitive' to light, the meaning is simply that light causes them to undergo certain changes or to be decomposed. It is their way of reacting to the stimulus received. And similarly, when we speak of a 'sensitive' balance or a 'sensitive' thermometer, we are indicating that these instruments are particularly apt to respond to circumstances by changes (movements of the balance-pans, for instance, or expansion of the mercury) and the sensitiveness will be so much the greater according as slighter external alterations, smaller differences in weight or temperature, are capable of producing corresponding changes in the apparatus. Though to my mind these analogies are not without interest or significance, I will not press them further since they hardly concern us here.

II. *Intelligence*

If we seek to discover an essential characteristic of intelligence, analogous to that which we have attempted to abstract from sensibility, we shall, I think, be led to conclude that this characteristic is knowledge. We shall see the reservations which have to be made in this definition and the criticisms which can be brought against it. Knowledge is, nevertheless, its characteristic fact.

What, then, in a fundamental sense, is knowledge? In the most general meaning of the term, it is the representation within ourselves of an external or internal reality, a representation which may help, which ought to help, if we regard the mind as a whole, to orientate our activity and to guide our conduct. Intelligence, indeed, constitutes a sort of preparation for action, by representing in us the reality towards which our activity will be directed. Thus it is that the knowledge of the topography of a town enables us to find our way to a given spot. Every fact of intelligence is thus a condition of our activity ; and associated with various other facts of the same kind, it enables us to perform very numerous and often very different actions. Hence our idea of water, the representation and knowledge we have of it, allows us to drink it, to go in a boat, to drive a locomotive, or to produce electricity ; and our knowledge of the properties of arsenic or bichloride of mercury permits us, similarly, to use the substance either as a remedy or as a poison.

Most of the facts which are labelled as intellectual phenomena readily admit of this conception of the intelligence. The evident function of perception, ideation and ratiocination, is to install within us a representation of reality, more or less accurate, symbolic, abstract or concrete, and to enable us to act upon that reality. There is no difficulty about this.

But difficulty may arise when we come to consider the play of the imagination. Imagination, as we know, does not invariably aim at or result in the representation of real things. Sometimes it imparts knowledge, because there are exact images and veracious combinations of images. Sometimes it terminates in knowledge, after a certain amount of error, for we have quite often to arrive at truth by way of fallacious hypotheses. But at other times, not only does the imagination fail to attain knowledge, but it does not wish to do so, and we do not wish it to do so : we deliberately guide it in another direction.

Neither partial error, involuntary error, nor intentional error can, however, essentially change the nature of intelligence. If perception, in so far as it relates to knowledge, is an intellectual fact, why should not hallucination, which occasionally simulates perception and is mistaken for it, also be one? And if my idea of a horse and my idea of a man are intellectual facts, what can my idea of a centaur be if not another intellectual fact? In such cases, whether it is a question of involuntary or intentional and deliberate errors, the function of the intelligence undergoes a partial transformation, a kind of deflection, but it preserves the same general characters. If it no longer represents a real world, it depicts a virtual world, an imaginary world, a world that is possible or impossible. It is always a representation, and in one sense always, subjectively at least, a form of knowledge.

Even in its most fantastic flights, the imagination is always an affirmation—often contradicted, checked, or suppressed by others, but still an affirmation. The proof of this is that when the 'reducers' disappear (insanity, dreams, absence of mind, etc.), belief in the reality of the facts reappears.[1] It is not enough to say, as some would do, that naturally the perception or the image is accompanied by a belief in the reality of the object; we must admit that the perception and the image are in themselves affirmations and beliefs—which *we* are able to apprehend as simple images without any other signification. If existence is a perception, it is a perception which the imagination imparts to everything that it presents to us. Everything that it represents, it represents as real, and it cannot do otherwise. It is other images and other ideas which arise to contradict the first and assert the unreality of their objects ; it is the mind as a whole which is normally able to settle the

[1] Cf. Taine, *De l'Intelligence*, Vol. I.

M

question ; but the negation always supposes at least an implicit affirmation.[1]

We admit, then, that perception and hallucination, correct or false ideas and images, true or false reasoning are all equally intellectual facts, since they are all affirmations and knowledge or pseudo-knowledge. As a consequence, we must widen our definition and say that intelligence consists essentially of knowledge, including in that term pseudo-knowledge, of the representation in us of a real world, possible or virtual or non-existent, but nevertheless affirmed by psychical facts similar in their general characters to those which affirm a real world. Furthermore, we must remember that it is very difficult and sometimes impossible to distinguish what is absolutely true in our knowledge, and that we can easily disbelieve our truest perceptions and most abstract ideas.

Intelligence has also as an essential character preparation for actions—the real or virtual guidance of conduct. We all know that accurate representation of the world—symbolically accurate at least—is a pre-eminent condition for successful and fruitful activity. Instances of this are innumerable, our lives are woven with them, from the sight of the fork which enables us to eat, to the astronomical discoveries that facilitate navigation. Ordinary life, industry, social relations, medicine, the whole of our activity, constantly prove the same thing.

What part does pseudo-knowledge play in this connection? There are many distinctions which we must make. Involuntary error continually gives rise to accidents, tragedies, calamities, disasters of every sort, in individual as in social life. At other times it paves the way for truth, and renders its advent possible :

[1] Perhaps it is not uninteresting to observe here that the words which denote a negation in French (*point, pas, mie*) have a positive sense on their own account, and that this positive sense appears (in the different forms of negation) to show their intensity. Thus, *point* denies more strongly than *pas*.

while we await the truth, this fills its place and behaves like it, so far as the mechanism of the action is concerned, if not when it comes to the evaluation of results. Alchemy, for example, and the history of medicine, would yield interesting facts in this connection. It appears, indeed, as though the unsatisfactory means of attending to wounds which were used in former times, and later on abandoned owing to the advance of medicine and observations which were more or less accurate, gave better results than the methods which replaced them and which were less effective in preserving the patient from unknown causes of infection. Sometimes again error and illusion seem to be essential to man. In many cases he can only live and be a social unit by the aid of erroneous beliefs, of insensate hopes that must inevitably be shattered, though they have thus enabled the life of the social organism to act and survive. Then again, there are voluntary illusions and workings of the imagination which appear to be in themselves their own objective. Voluntary illusions are sometimes utilized by the mind, and become elements of habit, conditions of the will. In art we see an illustration of their constant and systematic use. But apart from this case, which is rather special, though very common and exceedingly important,[1] the workings of imagination represent conditions of the will in the unreal world that they create, precisely in the same way as well-affirmed knowledge represents conditions of the will in the true world which it reveals.

III. *Affective Intelligence*

If sensibility is omnipresent in psychical life, the same applies to intelligence. The mind is intelligence, just as it is sensibility. Some sort of knowledge is manifest everywhere, and represents, implicitly or explicitly, a reality, correct or false. In the intellectual

---

[1] See, on this subject, the Author's *Mensonge de l'art.*

processes which are most highly specialized, this representative character is visible, patent, and dominant, but in others it is concealed, dissimulated, and subordinated. Nevertheless, the subjects of affective knowledge, and of knowledge through action, are interesting and important.

At the outset we may recall that an intellectual element is present in all the facts of consciousness, precisely in so far as they are conscious, that is to say, known to us; and that consequently they imply a knowledge and a representation of reality. So far as affective acts or volitions are conscious, consciousness being a knowledge, they are intellectual phenomena.

But more than this, the affective fact is in itself, at least in one of its aspects, a kind of knowledge, a representation of reality.

We must be careful not to confuse this essential intellectuality of feeling with its necessary and frequent connection with ideas and images. Our feelings are generally attended by images and ideas; an amorous passion scarcely exists without a representation of the person loved, without day-dreams and projects; nor an ambition without the idea of coveted advantages, and the means of acquiring them. These representations are essentially linked with the affective fact; if they are suppressed, there generally remains only a blind and stupid impulse. Consequently, we are almost continually recognizing intelligence in connection with feeling. But here I am claiming a far more essential identity of the intellectual fact with the affective fact which is generally regarded as solely dependent upon sensibility. Apart from ideas, images, and representations which are plainly intellectual, the affective fact persists in representing a part of a reality which may be external or internal, but is separate from itself. There is really an affective knowledge, an insecure, misleading knowledge, delusive even more often than the idea, but still a genuine and sometimes also a veridical knowledge, which without doubt may guide our conduct and instigate and direct our actions.

This is continually happening. The pain which we suffer from the prick of a pin, or from knocking against furniture in a dark room, is in itself a representation of the external world and of a part of its effects upon us. And without the intervention of ideas or reasoning, it directs our conduct and causes us to draw back our finger or to move forward more cautiously. The representation of the external world is here sufficiently plain for us to be able to state it in purely intellectual terms, in abstract propositions. But this operation is not at all necessary to enable knowledge to exist and be efficacious. The feeling alone suffices to represent the reality, and to direct actions. Some perceptions, of course, do take part in the representation; but it is obviously the affective side of the phenomenon which counts here, which informs us as to the qualities and happenings of the external world, and influences our conduct.

The pleasure we derive from the presence of a beloved person, even when this pleasure is not well understood by the intelligence or only half admitted, is a feeling which represents a whole series of external and internal realities, and in itself tends to determine our actions. Now, if we look for them, we can find reasons of an intellectual nature, enumerate the attractions of the person who fascinates us, specify the qualities of his or her mind and disposition, beauty or elegance, agreeableness or devotion. But all that is unnecessary, and the feeling sums up, synthesizes, and condenses into a single effective impression the long series of verifications and reasonings. It matters little whether the question be of love or of friendship. Assuredly Montaigne, had he desired, could have written at length to enlarge upon his " because it was he, because it was I ". And that might have been interesting; but, afterwards, would he have known his friend any better, would he have been more inclined to seek his company? That is not at all certain.

Every impression, every feeling, every affective fact, is thus in itself and by itself a sort of knowledge, a synthetic representation of varying exactitude, and it tends to facilitate actions and to direct the will. It is that too, but not that alone. On closer observation, we shall perceive that very often our representation of reality is not made up of clear ideas, of well-formulated and precisely-stated propositions, but rather of affective impressions, slight emotions, and feelings well defined or barely perceptible, but, nevertheless effective. There are also more indeterminate elements, of doubtful order, which cannot be positively classed as affective or intellectual, or neither the one nor the other; and this last series scales down into the unconscious, which we shall encounter again. In other words our internal representation of the world, if faithfully reproduced, would comprise more interjections than regularly-constructed phrases. It is not very often that we render an exact account, before acting, of the motives and facts upon which our procedure is based. When my pen becomes dry while I am writing, I do not say in a deliberate fashion : " There is no ink, that is why I cannot write ; I must therefore get some more, but my inkstand is over there, etc. "; I ascertain the fact, I have a slight feeling of irritation which sums up the situation, and I fill my pen without thinking about it, or almost without any thought.

Very often we could analyse the ideas, perceptions, recollections or considerations implicitly contained in our impression, and thus justify our conduct. But that is a social need, or a social duty, rather than a psychological necessity ; even unconscious knowledge is often enough.

Besides, the analysis is not always possible. Just now I remarked that Montaigne could have commented at length upon "because it was he, because it was

I ". And this is true, but it is probable that his analysis would not have exhausted the whole of his motives. His arguments, I should imagine, would certainly have omitted or disregarded reasons of sympathy that his heart could by no means forget. A mother does not very clearly understand why she loves her son, but her love synthesizes an infinite number of bonds which bind her to her child, without her perceiving them. It is an implicit knowledge of a number of individual facts, of her son's nature, of his relationship with herself, and, to some extent, of racial instincts and of social necessities.

Affective knowledge is infinitely more widespread than is commonly believed. It is mingled with the whole of our life. Whether reducible or not to intellectual formulæ, it is always of value. Sometimes it is ignored, though it may be in the right even when opposed to intelligence. For example, the first time we see a person, a priori antipathies and repulsions that it would be exceedingly difficult to explain or sudden and inexplicable sympathies, spring up within us. Occasionally we think it wiser to resist these impressions, but prolonged experience may justify them and humiliate the reasoning judgment before feeling. We had disregarded the knowledge which lay concealed in feeling and was accessible to us only through that agency.

Thus valuable instinctive warnings may be fruitlessly expended upon us ; we do not guess their value because there is no precise verification and clear reasoning in their workings. Not all the arguments founded upon " the impulses of feeling " and " the needs of the heart " are absurd and false. Pascal's saying about the reasons of the heart that reason does not know betrays a good observer and a wise philosopher. But it has been singularly abused, like all sentimental arguments, by being introduced where it was not relevant. Nothing is easier, indeed, than to invoke a pretended feeling in support of anything we wish to prove, to mistake a desire or a vague aspiration for a reality, and to erect the scaffolding of a world-system upon a few paltry personal impressions, or even one of those collective feelings which have neither the meaning nor the scope that is assigned to them.

Affective knowledge would require a still more rigorous and detailed criticism than intellectual knowledge. Unfortunately, the study of it is more difficult, and requires more patience, acumen, and detailed care; but the practice of analysis may lead to a better understanding of affective knowledge as well as to a discovery, in many instances, of its rational grounds. There are instinctive impressions whose value can be thus determined. It is also possible in certain cases for us to discover or conjecture the origin, or probable origin, of the individual or collective impression which appears to contain implicit knowledge and tends to direct activity. The knowledge of the source of an impression may often inform us as to its value. This is the case, for example, when a superficial or accidental resemblance of one person to another prompts in us feelings towards the one similar to those which we experienced for the other.

Affective knowledge, moreover, is more fallacious and less truly instructive than reasoned and more obviously intellectual knowledge. It can distort reality, or so disregard it as to leave man powerless or drive him into dangerous errors and regrettable actions.

I say man. Perhaps it is different with animals. The relative security of instinct has so often been contrasted with the relative inadequacy of intelligence that I need not dwell upon it. And instinct is, perhaps, in one of its principal aspects and in certain cases, a kind of affective knowledge; in other instances it may be merely unconscious knowledge. The wonders of the instinct of *Sphex*, which J. H. Fabre has made deservedly famous, are widely known. There we have an example of implicit knowledge which baffles us, even if it has not the inevitable certainty which the entomologist of Sérignan describes.

It is easy enough to recognize in man distinct signs of instincts and affective knowledge. But civilization and socialization have in many respects distorted these instincts and made the knowledge uncertain. Thus man's inclination causes him to take pleasure in certain beverages and foods which are injurious to him. Nevertheless, even in man, repugnance is in some degree representative of danger, and is often equivalent to a knowledge of the noxious character of the thing which excites disgust. A similar instinct keeps us aloof from certain persons and gives us a sort of warning of danger in their presence. It is an analogous instinct which informs us that we shall prosper in such and such an undertaking or study, and aptitude is often disclosed by an attraction towards, or an enthusiasm for a particular occupation.

If we consider the enormous part played in man's life by semi-automatic activity, which is not reasoned and is manifested by impressions and affective signs, we shall see that affective knowledge (as well as unconscious knowledge) is extremely widespread and of capital importance. In our social relations, as in the guidance of our individual conduct, it is constantly intervening. I have mentioned the instinctive likings and antipathies, appetites and distastes, vocations and repulsions. All these facts implicitly contain an incalculable number of condensed items of knowledge, which intellectual analysis can sometimes disentangle, if it takes the trouble. If we wished to make a fairly complete review of affective knowledge, other facts would have to be added. It is to affective knowledge that we must refer those half-instincts, those synthetic and appreciative sentiments whose intellectual side cannot be disregarded—'tact' in social relations, literary and general æsthetic 'taste', and even the moral 'conscience'. Such knowledge and judgments cannot always be reduced to precise intellectual formulæ; they are rather states of feeling which enlighten and direct.

In such cases, intellectual analysis is even repugnant. The feeling affirms, but it does not prove its assertions by regular and formal arguments. A person affirms that this picture is beautiful, that that individual was right or wrong to behave as he did, that murder is always a culpable action. You ask him why, and he shrugs his shoulders; if you insist, he says that one feels it to be so; if you don't, you are wrong, and so much the worse for you. Everyone knows the horror manifested by some people, in whom affective knowledge is preponderant, at the analysis and discussion of æsthetics or morals. It was they who invented the proverb, *De gustibus* . . ., which, like all proverbs, must not be taken too seriously. Analysis can, in fact, in a great many cases, vindicate or condemn a taste, an inspiration, or any affective knowledge.

Common sense, good sense, a certain logical sense, have still to be considered in connection with affective knowledge. A peculiar impression warns us that some fact is improbable, some argument unsound, or it may tell us the contrary. Here again we experience attractions and dislikes which decide the greater part of our beliefs and opinions. "It follows, of course"; "So-and-so lacks good sense"; "it isn't common sense"; such are the expressions, constantly repeated, of our affective and instinctive opinions. If we have the habit and feeling for close reasoning, a *petitio principii*, any break or flaw whatever in the strict chain of ideas, immediately gives us a characteristic impression, a sort of uneasiness, an unæsthetic feeling, which tells us at once that the reasoning is erroneous even before we analyse it.

Whatever use may be made of analysis—and for my part I would willingly allow it a large part—it is important to recognize that it is not all-sufficing, and that an exaggeration of its role would arrest thought itself. How should we manage without 'taste', 'tact', conscience, good sense, and logicality? Beyond question, they often deceive man ; but analysis, observation, and reasoning deceive him also. Can we conceive that we ought to reduce all life to intellectual formulæ, to observe each impression minutely and reason about it ; that we ought to infer and deduce unceasingly in order to regulate every instant of our behaviour towards others, to appreciate a piece of verse or a symphony, to judge of the worth of an action, or to accept or reject an insignificant truth? Life would become impossible —happily, perhaps! On all occasions observation, analysis, and reasoning are necessary to us and we must not place a blind trust in affective knowledge : we must know how to rectify it, contradict it, and remain sceptical before it, how to illuminate, direct, and amend our intellectual instincts ; but we must not pretend to do without affective knowledge.

How far this affective knowledge can reason, it is exceedingly difficult to ascertain. We have all known cases in which intellectual instinct was right, as opposed to reason—for the reasoning reason is a clumsy faculty, almost as clumsy as it is useful and necessary. We are sometimes impressed with the sagacity of the instinct, and with the teachings it conveys about men and things. What we learn from animals in this respect is marvellous and inexplicable. Man's instinct, enfeebled and disordered, is still capable of surprising actions, which have not perhaps been sufficiently investigated. There seem to be cases of singular penetration, which it would be interesting to study more attentively than we have hitherto done. Telepathy and divination, if there is anything genuine in them, as certain facts seem to suggest, may induce us to suspect the existence of a mode of knowledge similar to affective knowledge and instinctive knowledge. But the whole subject is still too little understood to be discussed at length here.

Affective knowledge varies greatly with the individual. Everybody has remarked that some minds are more instinctive, more impulsive, and that their opinions have the air of being felt rather than considered and debated. They have no liking for minute inquiry, patient analysis, or sceptical consideration. Woman, still more than man, appears generally to rely upon the affective knowledge which is dominant within her. There is doubtless a connection between training, education, and the type of knowledge. Affective knowledge is necessarily more widespread among unlettered and ignorant people, whose minds have not been trained by complicated methods. This gives them certain disadvantages, but, on some occasions, a certain superiority. Other minds, on the contrary, can be induced to admit nothing without serious reflection ; the affective impression, the sympathy or antipathy felt for a particular idea, is for them only a starting-point, not their ultimate destination, and another instinct impels them to mistrust it. Their principal concern is to produce an even balance between their various kinds of knowledge, and to combine them so that one controls and rectifies the other.

I have already drawn attention to the qualitative variation of affective knowledge, that is of instincts, in different individuals. It varies as greatly as the power of analysing and reasoning. But it is not distributed upon the same plan. Sometimes affective knowledge is good, but is accompanied by notable incapacity in analysis and reasoning ; sometimes it is the reverse ; or, again, the good and the bad may draw the mind in different directions at the same time. There are people whose feelings are awkward, and even rather stupid. Their affective knowledge is erroneous, and readily leads them to do foolish things ; it represents reality in a transfigured form, and frequently influences or perverts observation, judgment, and reasoning. These latter are always under its subjection and guidance—they are its accompaniment and interpretation, so to speak. They assist it in turning conduct into perilous and disastrous channels. The illusions to which sexual love, maternal love, and even friendship and esteem are liable, are no longer taken into account. " I love this person, therefore she has such and such a quality ", is very nearly the intellectual formula which represents the claims of the affective understanding. Laughable as it may appear to a reasoning person it is not necessarily absurd. It contains just as much truth as the statement that we only like persons endowed with such and such a virtue. Something of the kind really takes place, and in a very sound and clear mind, instinctive sympathy is often a sufficient guarantee of harmony between the two natures, and of the presence of certain qualities in the person who has been able to inspire sympathy. We reason in much the same way when we say : " I like mathematics, so I shall probably do well at it "; and, indeed, in a healthy mind, the vocation is determined by aptitude (or else it is speedily discouraged, and does not persist). Or, again, " I ate this food with relish, so I shall probably digest it well ";—which is generally true. In matters of art our reasoning is always very much like this. " This sonnet is beautiful because it pleases me ; that opera is good, for I enjoyed seeing it performed "; and thence we go headlong on the downward path to such examples of criticism as " Give me a melodrama in which Marguerite wept ", or " If it makes you cry it can't be wrong ".

Even these formulæ may have a particle of truth in them, which it would be interesting to bring to light if space allowed. In philosophy, we discover, plainly enough, an analogous formula : " I love life, so I shall live for ever ", "I aspire to justice, therefore justice will be realized, etc.", which comes near to " I am hungry, therefore I shall always have something to eat ". Even this last formula, with certain alterations, presents an unquestionable reality. " I am hungry " does not imply that I shall always have something to eat, but it does indicate, since it specially concerns a need which is common to all living beings, that there is food in the world, and that beings in a normal situation eat from time to time. Similarly, the love of justice or of happiness doubtless proves that there is in society, at least in certain respects, something which may be regarded as happiness or justice.

But in many cases this instinct is fallacious, and in certain persons affective knowledge is unsound. ' Misfits ' are the people whose calling is founded upon a mistaken affective understanding, always excepting those who owe their failure to external circumstances, such as some calamity, or to the public's want of comprehension. Too many, beguiled by the pleasures of the palate, take a delight in harmful foods and drinks. And the sexual instinct has led astray countless lovers who, without taking anything else into account, have tried to draw from it conclusions which it is incapable of supplying.

Other minds, on the contrary, are distinguished by a rare sureness of instinct; their affections are intelligent —clear-sighted, we might say. They feel reality rather than consciously observe or reason about it. A safe instinct seems to warn and direct them, to represent reality to them—a reality which is sometimes hidden and profound. But even by privileged beings this characteristic is not invariably possessed—for example, sexual love is seldom clear-sighted and rational. This, it would seem, is the passion which has most power to deceive man—and woman—which most effectually disguises reality from them, and most easily seduces them to folly and misfortune.

And this leads us to inquire as to the causes of these errors in instinct, and of the imperfections of the affective understanding.

It is especially in man that these illusions of instinct and feeling are frequent and serious, and it is in him that they can be most easily examined. Probably, therefore, they are connected with his special nature, with the qualities which give him a place apart among animals. The chief of these qualities is that man is *an animal who has not yet accepted his life;* who is not adapted to the principal condition of his existence, namely society; and who is incessantly occupied with transforming the conditions of his existence and his manner of submitting to them and of submitting them to himself, without ever having been able to find his equilibrium.

Man inherited from his animal ancestors a certain number of instincts which were relatively trustworthy. It would seem that some of them are better preserved by tribes less civilized than ourselves. But by incessantly complicating his social life and by placing himself in novel and unusual conditions, man has modified the circumstances in which his instincts must be exercised to such an extent that instinct, somewhat inflexible by nature, has been unable to transform itself as it should have done. If we adopted the seductive and dubious hypothesis which regards instinct as hereditary custom, we should understand that new habits have not been able to organize themselves and take deep root in our being. But all this remains exceedingly hypothetical, and the theory of instinct, as it was accepted some thirty years ago, is faced by great difficulties.

Even the instinct of animals does not always resist changes of environment, especially what may be called social environment. Man is able to pervert the affective understanding of his humble friends; it is not surprising that his own has often become weaker. Taste and scent inform the dog as to the value for him of the grasses he finds in the meadows, but not as to the effects of wine, for example. Man also tries to make use of his instincts, in order to gain knowledge which they cannot supply. Alcoholism, drunkenness, and various maladies thus testify to errors of instinct, and especially of taste; but equally love bears witness to the errors in which the sexual instinct ends when we attempt to derive from it indications different from that which it has to give. In a healthy being, the inclination of the senses promises pleasure in sexual union, and perhaps also the continuance of the race in good conditions (since normal desire is more readily directed towards young persons of healthy appearance). But it is absurd to use it as a guide in seeking qualities of character, mind, or any social gifts which will assure the happiness of an enamoured pair during the whole of their common life. Nevertheless, it is customary to do so. Undoubtedly the sexual instinct is complicated by being associated with a great many different feelings, such as esteem and sympathy, but those feelings are not always trustworthy, and the ardour of the sexual instinct continually interferes with their operation. Nothing is more common than to attach to the person marked out by the sexual instinct characters of heart and mind of which he or she is destitute. And often it is this which is called love. In the same way, it is the complicated nature of social life and its transmutations which have produced the majority of the affective errors that have obstructed man's intelligence, and begotten or sustained most of his religious and metaphysical illusions. Man has ended by mistaking his preferences for the rules of present and future reality. Bossuet in his day observed that this is a very dangerous proceeding. In religion as in philosophy, in ethics as in politics, even in science and social life and throughout his whole existence, man has suffered cruelly in this way, without making any great attempt to mend his ways. Then again we may observe how frequently a man will be satisfied with a political system for some moral reason, or from some obscure instinct ; he will instantly decide that it is more conducive than any other to the well-being of his country.

Is it possible to correct the errors of the affective understanding or to contrive to prevent them from being hurtful? It has become a kind of psychological commonplace that intellect is always vanquished in a contest with feeling. Still, it must be admitted that in such a strife the intelligence on its side is also strengthened by feeling : and that reasoning does not always remain unproductive. When it is properly employed, moreover, it has the effect of mobilizing the feelings, of calling them up in order that they may be of assistance, and occasionally of making them pass over from one side to the other. There are plenty of people who upon occasion have stopped doing something which pleased them, because they have become aware of its attendant disadvantages, through the advice of others or through their own reflection. Analysis can sometimes be practised with success, though obviously it requires a certain application and skill. A lover will scarcely be discouraged by sermonizing, even of the most discreet kind, or by attempts to show him upon æsthetic grounds that his idol is less beautiful than he believes. But it is not at all unprecedented, I think, for scandal and calumny to separate friends and even lovers. It is not impossible, then, to work upon a feeling. This is no place for investigating the form and rules of such action, and I confine myself to the few indications which have been given in the course of this hasty survey of the matter, in which the general psychological aspect of the phenomena has been our especial interest.

IV. *Knowledge in Will*

While seeking intelligence in the feelings, we have discovered it also in the will, and in all forms of activity. The instincts of which we have just spoken constantly intermingle decisions with impressions and feelings— which, as we shall see, are also decisions in and of themselves. What was said of one of them may be said of the others.

In every volition and every decision, whatever order it may belong to, there is also a knowledge or pseudo-

N

knowledge of reality. To will an action and even simply to act implies a knowledge, a belief, and a whole system of knowledge and beliefs which may very well assume any form other than those of distinct ideas and conscious judgments. Sometimes, also, our clear ideas and conscious judgments are contradictory to the implicit knowledge and beliefs which make us act and which are just as real and often stronger than the first. Our decisions by themselves contain, no less, a true or false representation of reality. A reflex action itself, even an unconscious reflex, signifies a knowledge of some detail at least of the external world. When our pupil dilates because the light decreases, the reason is that a certain knowledge of external events has reached us, even though we may not have noticed them or been conscious of them in any way. To take a remedy is to affirm and evince one's faith in the efficacy of that remedy. The affirmation may be feigned, the belief may be rejected by the conscious and analytical intelligence, but none the less it is an affirmation and a knowledge, or at least a pseudo-knowledge, a kind of idea which is itself a fact of the intellectual order. A decision, reflex, automatic, affective or considered, and assuming the form of an act of volition, is invariably in itself an affirmation, and is always an indication of some intellectual influence.

Moreover, action is always regarded as a means of suggesting belief, that is knowledge or pseudo-knowledge accepted by the mind. This is because it already implies a knowledge, which tends, according to the ordinary working of systematic association, to obtrude upon the rest of the mind, the feelings as well as the conscious intelligence, so as to make it appear true. This fact is so well known that there is no need to attempt to prove it. We need merely recall hypnotic suggestion, subjects in whom ideas and feelings can be aroused by causing them to make some gesture or adopt some attitude ; the liar who by force of repetition is finally deceived by his own lying; the particles of truth contained in the Lange-James theory concerning the emotions which are always accompanied by certain ideas and beliefs. We might also recall Pascal's advice to unbelievers : " Follow the way in which they began : that is, doing everything as if they believed, making use of holy water, going to mass, etc. This will naturally lead you too to believe and will blunt your senses." From all these facts it is evident that volition and activity include knowledge, and that they are an affirmation. The knowledge is implicit, and the affirmation may be more or less sincere, that is to say, more or less accepted by the mind, though it may remain in the form of an independent psychical element. But we see that often the mere act, or its systematic repetition, suffices to develop the idea, to give it its distinctive form and also to impress it upon the rest of the mind and cause it to be accepted as true. The intellectual side of activity is manifested in this process; it is liberated and affirmed, and its efficacy and power established.

Furthermore, volition and activity in general sometimes reveal more clearly than the conscious intelligence the deep-seated beliefs and hereditary opinions which lie imprisoned but potent in the mind. How many people act in opposition to their avowed opinions, to those which they themselves imagine they hold ! Often, undoubtedly, they do so because behaviour which was in accordance with these opinions would entail some inconvenience. In that case, their mind is divided, their personality is dissociated, and their practical affirmations contradict their theoretical affirmations. But often such inconsistency arises from the fact that the beliefs which they imagine to be theirs have only lightly touched their mind and rested on its surface. They are like a borrowed garment, cut to the fashion of the day, or acquired under strong transient influences, while other opinions—correct or erroneous—continue to live in the depths of the mind, to guide an important side of conduct, and to affirm their presence by significant actions. "Is the belief which never shows itself in action a sincere belief?" We can always ask this question, and also whether the negation that permits action is sincere. Doubt or negation must frequently be the reply.

Volition or activity is, moreover, always an affirmation whose nature, meaning, and scope must be discussed in every case. The person who acts, if considered as a whole, may not believe in everything that his action implies—prudence, hypocrisy, humanity, even the desire to believe—but the action itself knows (perfectly or imperfectly) and affirms ; and its affirmation is contagious and tends to encroach.

Thus everywhere in the mind we find the essential character of intelligence, and more or less conscious knowledge ; the representation within ourselves of a reality, a possibility, external or internal—a representation normally destined to permit, prepare and direct action. We have not thought it necessary to consider this last character here, since it is very obvious in the intellectual side of volition.

V. *Volition as a Decisive Synthesis in Intelligence and in Affective Facts*

The essential character of volition is that it constitutes a decisive synthesis, establishes a man's way of life and his attitude of mind, and sets in motion a series of actions or manifold transformations which proceed to unfold themselves, according to circumstances, in conformity with what it has decreed. It is a creation.

This is evident for the most characteristic facts of the will, or those which are generally regarded as such. The man who, after doubts, reflections and long consideration, finally takes up a position, synthesizes in an act of volition the motives of action which have brought him to this decision. He relates the feelings and ideas that he has singled out to all the psychical elements whose activity will bring about the accomplishment of the desired action. At the same time, he thrusts aside tendencies, desires, and ideas which were opposed to his decision ; adverse beliefs and feelings are weakened or disappear, and the series of actions, organized in accordance with the voluntary decision, unfolds itself in systematic fashion.

But between clear volitions and all the other cases of activity lie such an infinity of shades that we are not justified in drawing a very rigid line of demarcation. The character of decisive synthesis, which marks volition, is also encountered in what may be called affective activity. When we act without any particular hesitation, without visible deliberation, under the influence of a feeling, the synthesis of the motives, ideas, impressions and motor elements is effected in a slightly different manner—more swiftly, more easily ; but it is not very different. In fact, we constantly say that we 'intended' an action which has been spontaneously accomplished, without any struggle and without the active intervention of the personality as a whole, or of the psychical elements more especially representing it. And in all forms of activity, whether volitional, automatic, instinctive or even reflex, we can always observe this essential character of will, as being a decisive and systematic synthesis. It is impossible, starting from the most characteristic volition and descending step by step to the reflex, to discover a precise line of demarcation where the essential nature of activity is changed.

But this character of decisive synthesis which marks volition is also encountered in all psychical facts. Certainly it would be incorrect to assert that all mental phenomena are facts of volition—although that has been maintained : we merely say that volition is omnipresent in the mind, just as intelligence and sensibility are.

Volition, over and above the principal character already recognized, implies a certain newness in the action, something analogous to creative activity or genius. In this sense it is opposed, very sharply in certain cases, to routine, instinct and habit. But, on the one hand, this inventive character is not peculiar to volition properly so-called, for it is also encountered in intellectual and affective facts ; and, on the other hand, even within the domain of volition we find nothing but nuances and combinations. There is no act of will which is detached from every form of instinctive or reflex activity, and similarly there is no act of instinct or routine which in itself exactly reproduces another in every detail of its conditions, its elements, and the activity of its elements. In this sense, also, volition is omnipresent.

But passing from the sphere which is usually regarded as peculiar to will, we find that in intellectual and affective facts volition is represented by all the features which most essentially characterize it.

A short time ago there was considerable discussion as to the relations of belief and will, and of will and error. One much debated thesis introduced freedom into judgment. Ardently sustained, and opposed with similar ardour, it gave way to other controversies. I do not wish to revive that issue here, interesting though it was, and I will, therefore, put aside for the moment the question of free will. But of the whole theory I retain one very real fact upon which it claimed to be based. The adoption of a belief is an occurrence which may well be compared with a voluntary action. The deliberation, the examination of motives, the weighing of reasons on both sides, are alike in both cases. Intellectual deliberation also admits of its doubts and anxieties, sometimes even its troubles. The decision itself is analogous in volition and in the adoption of the belief. It is a synthesis which makes a new combination of elements that were

previously scattered. The decision embodies in the
mind a doctrine, a system of ideas, a creed, instead of
giving it practical activity, but the annexation, the
assimilation by the ego is the same in the two cases,
and displays the same general characters ; similarly
it is an accepted choice, a constructive synthesis which
is imposed, involving the rejection, the casting off, the
dissociation, or even the disappearance of the unaccept-
able elements. Jouffroy's night of doubt, which we
mentioned before, certainly gives the impression of a
crisis of will as well as of an intellectual crisis : it is
both at the same time. A conversion appears to be
a decision of the will, as well as a transformation of the
intelligence. And the fact of the ego accepting a new
doctrine, and making it its own, is entirely identical, in
every essential respect, with a volition.

If we look more closely into the matter, we shall
discern in every mental operation, upon a reduced scale,
and also with some secondary differences, an indisput-
able equivalent of an act of volition. Any opinion
whatsoever, even an idea or a perception, from the very
fact that it is accepted by the mind, always shows a
decisive character which determines, for a more or less
considerable period and over a more or less extensive
field, the attitude of the mind, or at least of some of its
elements, or even of one alone, if we wish to go so far
and take it to its logical conclusion. Number here has
nothing to do with the matter, and the phenomenon
remains the same, whatever its scale. All that has
been said with regard to the acceptance of a fact is
equally applicable to its rejection. To reject an idea,
to efface an image, is as much a decision as to accept it.
In this case certain secondary characters of the
voluntary decision are undoubtedly weakened, but we
cannot claim that even these entirely disappear. A
distinct perception is not always formed at the outset ;

the mind wavers, it fails to distinguish, labours and struggles, and when perception is at last established, combining the dispersed elements, it claims a sort of victory. This happens, for instance, when we try to recognize a person or an object from some distance away, when we wish to read an inscription which is too far off, or to decipher a difficult piece of handwriting.

It is often the same with the revival of an image : it is produced after a voluntary effort, resembling that which determines a volition, and in itself, indeed, it is a kind of volition, which determines the form of the mind, and invokes and co-ordinates the various elements, under the impulse of an accepted desire. The cases in which the image and the perception do not eventually take shape are for the most part cases of faint desires, exactly like contradictory volitions or mere desires of the will, incapable of leading to anything, such as we notice frequently in the course of practical life.

In such cases, the process of making up the mind does not, of course, assume the same importance as a volition involving the whole of life and imposing a definite course upon it, or as one involving the adoption of a creed which will probably disorganize in various ways the entire intellectual life, as well as the affective and practical. But unimportant though it may be, it is none the less a fixation, either of the mind as a whole or of certain of its elements. The most fugitive fact always has its own settled form, which is different from that of any other ; I would even say its ' definitive ' form however shortlived it may be. If it really existed, it existed as one . special thing, not as something different. The advent of this form, this decisive synthesis which exists at a given instant, which is itself and nothing else, is almost the infinitesimal element of will.

Or we can put it in a different way and say that it is an ' elementary ' will. In this case the mind as a whole does not always intervene, at least in an appreciable way. At the most, it probably exercises a control, which is not without importance, enabling it to attribute to itself many facts in which it does not take a very evident or active part, but which none the less pertain to it : somewhat as the manager of a factory ascribes to himself the things produced by the workmen under him, or as a general ascribes to himself the deeds of soldiers whom he need not know individually nor follow in all their evolutions.

Here, therefore, not only the mind but also its elements must be considered. All the minor happenings in the mind represent the more or less independent and, occasionally, rebellious activity of its constituent elements. They are, from this point of view, so many little elementary volitions, more or less submissive to a general will, which has created them and still directs them, or merely allows them to operate, while holding them under its control. Sometimes they also indicate an insurrection of these elementary wills against other elementary wills, or against the general will.[1] But in all these cases, the essential characters which concern us here undergo very little change.

The type of these elementary wills can be recognized in twitchings of the body, and in certain pathological facts such as those which have been ascribed to larval epilepsy. A man suddenly begins to make incoherent gestures or performs some trifling action, and then resumes his previous occupation without remembering anything. In the normal state facts of this kind are not uncommon, although generally less characteristic. Many people have little eccentricities, familiar mannerisms, of which they are unaware. The tendency exists in them, and at the same time outside them. In the intellectual sphere, similar phenomena are also produced. An image, an idea, occurs unexpectedly, without one's knowing why ; it floats an instant in the mind, and disappears without leaving an appreciable trace. But

[1] For the independent life of the elements of the mind, see the author's *l'Activité mentale*, Part I.

at the moment when these phenomena are produced, they also are decisive syntheses, elementary volitions of a sort, which combine into a precise attitude certain elements of the mind. They are to the main volition what the few elements they fix for an instant are to the mind as a whole and to the continuation of its life.

What we have just said of intellectual facts naturally applies to feelings also. A *grande passion*, however involuntary it may be in one sense and so far as appearances are concerned, includes also, when it is affirmed, the essential characters of an action of will. Whether love is born suddenly, or is organized and accepted little by little, the moment when it distinctly assumes its own character, when it dawns upon the mind as admitted love, is, like volition, a decisive synthesis. This synthesis also determines the orientation of the mind and proceeds to control its direction. It combines tendencies, desires, impressions, ideas, into a systematic whole, and it dismisses others, repelling, disorganizing, or annihilating them. It goes on developing into long series of ideas, feelings, and actions, and expresses the nature of the mind and its personal reaction in given circumstances. These are just the characteristics of a voluntary decision. It is the same with ambition, or with any passion whatsoever.

In many cases, passion and will almost coalesce, volition being little more than the logical consequence, the spontaneous manifestation of the passion that is acknowledged and accepted. A passion also appears not infrequently as the expression of will. "I have vowed to live and die for love", said Musset. Passion in reality is the expression of the personality itself, of an important part of the organized ego, partly unconscious, often stronger and more intimate than the conscious ego we know. How could we separate the ambition of Napoleon from his will, or the love of Musset or the intellectual passion of Spinoza from theirs?

But why then are volition and passion or feeling sometimes represented as being opposed? Feeling, it may be said, may quite possibly be a condition of will, but it is certainly not the result of will. We will a certain action because we feel a certain desire, but we do not will to have the desire; it is born in us apart from our will, sometimes against our will. It is true that our volitions depend upon our desires; yet what are these desires but the expression and consequence of the tendencies, desires, and ideas that existed before them, in the circumstances which life presented? And hence they also are a kind of decision of the mind, an unconscious or only half-conscious decision, but a decision all the same. We might gradually travel back step by step throughout a whole human life, as far as the formation of the individual. And from that point of view life would seem to us like a long unfolding of manifold decisions, organizing themselves into an incomplete and confused system. There is no need for me to inquire here whether these decisions might have been in certain comparatively rare cases, or in all cases, or in no case, different from what they actually were. I do not think that the solution of the problem of free will is indispensable to our present investigation.

We have still to consider the relatively independent activity of the psychic elements and their systems. Passion sometimes appears to be opposed to will, because it checks other desires, because it comes into collision with antagonistic tendencies, supported in certain cases by the conscious ego. This is because the conscious ego is only one part of our actual personality. It is, in such cases, like a king deposed from power by a rebel chief who has succeeded in mobilizing the principal forces of the country. In the name of his official authority, the monarch asserts that the country desires him to subdue his adversaries, but the leader of the rebels wills otherwise, and his will is also the will of the country, more so even than that of the king.

Similarly, the superficial ego, which has lost the habit of directing the deep and hidden forces of the mind, or which does not know how to lay hold of them or has even been unaware of them all the time, may find itself assailed by them. Its will may then be different from theirs, but those unknown and oppressed forces also have a will, and their will is likewise the will of the organism and the mind. The conflicts between passion and will are invariably struggles between tendencies and between wills.

From important affective facts such as passions and great and powerful feelings, we can descend to the most trivial, taking up again the considerations which were developed in connection with ideas. It seems, therefore, unnecessary to elaborate them. The affective fact in all its variations of degree appears as a decision.

Thus everywhere in the mind we encounter will, as everywhere we encounter intelligence and sensibility. The mind is sensibility, it is knowledge, it is active will. No doubt in speaking thus we change the ordinary meaning of the words a little, but this is necessary, since the ordinary meaning of the words or too narrow an interpretation of them does not permit us to arrive at a satisfactory conception of the mind and its divisions. Both lead inevitably to confusion and error. It is also justified in that we have endeavoured to abstract from the usual meaning of the words the essential characters which they denote.

Feeling, intelligence, and will are not, therefore, clearly delimited and separate groups of facts, any more than they are the products of three distinct metaphysical faculties. They are, in fact, diffused in every part of the mind : there is no fragment of mental life, however insignificant, which does not exhibit all three of them at work. But in certain cases we are more impressed by the character of activity ; in others the character of knowledge is more obvious; and, lastly, in others sensibility is more readily apparent to the observer.

VI. *Epilogue*

It remains for us to examine the reasons which have brought about this result and have led the observer to select one aspect of the psychical fact in order to characterize and describe the fact itself.

We have undoubtedly been in the habit of considering too exclusively the activity of the entire personality, while neglecting the particular activity and the relatively independent life of its elements. Thus we have regarded as facts of sensibility all those in which the mind, viewed as a whole, was seen to be activated by an external, or internal cause—sensations, feelings, emotions, etc. We have classed under intelligence all those that represent for the conscious mind the real world and the imaginary world, with their combinations and dissociations—perceptions, ideas, judgments, reasonings, analysis, abstraction, etc. ; and, finally, we have referred to the will those which point to the activity of the person as a whole. Naturally the classifications arrived at in this way have been somewhat vague and defective ; nor was any other result possible. Nevertheless, in certain respects, they square fairly well with the theories which make reflex action the type of psychical life ; and these theories can in their turn be reconciled with different views.

No importance has been attached to the general fact that the phenomena of sensibility and intelligence are also kinds of volition, and that, to a varying extent, intelligence is present in sensibility and sensibility in intelligence: nor has it even been noticed sufficiently. Every fact was taken, not for what it really was in itself, but for its function approximately recognized in the working of the mind as a whole. We may recall here what happens when a magnet is broken in pieces—

not of course that we would identify the two series of phenomena, or even claim for them essential and fundamental resemblances. The magnet, in its original form, has a positive and a negative pole. If we break it, each fragment still possesses its two poles, and so on for every further division. Similarly we can, on a somewhat over-simplified level, observe in the mind a sensibility, an intelligence, and a will. But if, instead of considering the mental ensemble, we consider its elements, each of these still exhibits the same qualities and the same powers ; and the elements of the elements, again, possess the same properties. Only there is no need for the mind to be broken up before sensibility, intelligence, and will can appear in its elements and become perceptible.

But a consideration of the mind as a whole could not lead to a precise estimate of psychical facts or to a strict classification—a classification which could never have been got at along the lines which were being followed. When we range an idea among intellectual facts and a decision among the facts of will, we are doubtless making an approximation sufficient for the requirements of daily life. Yet even this would not be free from inconveniences were not certain reservations understood. But where other facts are concerned, difficulties spring up much more easily. Sensation and perception, for example, are at once, even from the narrow traditional point of view we are considering at the moment, facts of intelligence and facts of sensibility. And though we may seem to avoid the difficulty by restricting sensibility to the appearance of pleasure and pain, this position is distinctly weak, very narrow, and scarcely tenable. Pleasure and pain are certainly indications of sensibility, and are closely linked to it, but they are not sufficient to constitute and define it.

On the other hand, although sensibility, intelligence, in so far as representation is concerned, and will or activity are encountered in every psychological phenomenon, it is more useful in many circumstances to emphasize sometimes one of these aspects of the same fact and sometimes another. Pleasure and pain, for instance, certainly represent within us some external or internal reality, but this reality is difficult to recognize with any precision. The process often requires long experience and patient analysis. But that pleasure generally attracts us and pain tends to repel us, that these two opposed facts are the most apt to set the machinery of our mind in motion, above all that they make us perceive there a change corresponding to external or internal circumstances — this is plainly apparent, more easily verifiable, and perhaps more frequently useful to realize. Whether they are in fact a sign of an active reaction of our ego, is neither easy to determine, nor of very much importance in the greater part of practical life. And therefore we tend to connect pleasure and pain solely with sensibility, without paying much attention to their intellectual aspect or thinking of them as active and partly voluntary reactions.

Thus in every case we ought to be able to discover some reason based upon utility or convenience, which has caused a particular psychical fact to be placed in a particular one of the three great commonly accepted divisions. And the primary reason, whose importance has induced me to call attention to it separately, the consideration of the part played by a fact in the totality of mental life, is itself a reason of utility and convenience.

Naturally, the framework of faculties or groups of phenomena so constructed could not remain unchanged, inflexible, and solid. It had either to break or bend. And in fact, although psychologists do not appear to have paid sufficient attention to the fact, this framework has been stretched, twisted, and broken by the friends of unity, simple synthesis, and generalization on the one hand, and on the other by observers whose experience has been ceaselessly transformed by an unstable reality, and has continuously presented to them different reasons,

of convenience and expediency, little noticed by the
generality of mankind. I have already had occasion to
describe some of these experiences. They have not all
been realized in the domain of scientific psychology. The
notion of intellectual sensibility, for example, is utilized
more especially by literary men and critics, and I merely
allude here to the attempts which have been made to
refer the essential basis of the mind either to sensibility,
to 'representations', which are rather of an intellectual
order, to activity, or to the will. The reason is not only
that we are undoubtedly sometimes compelled to admit
that sensibility is encountered in intelligence and will,
intelligence in sensibility, volition in intelligence, and
so on ; but the activity of the mental elements, especially
the most important of them, the most complex and the
best organized, is occasionally evident enough to make
perceptible the sensibility, intelligence, and activity
proper to every one of those psychic systems. We are
often rather surprised to find that the same person
exhibits intelligent aims and blind desires, active
passions and somewhat sluggish feelings, some tendencies that are sentimental and others that remain
torpid, indifferent, difficult to arouse. This compels us
to speak of sensitive intelligence or of intelligent passions,
and inclines us to look for the characteristics of the
qualities of large groups of psychic facts in a single fact.

None the less, provided there is a clear understanding on the matter, it proves convenient and
sometimes valuable, as well as perfectly legitimate, to
consider the sensibility, intelligence, and will of the
individual as a whole, and not in single elements ; to
take some fact which involves many others and observe
it for a moment, under one of its aspects only, noticing
merely that which particularly interests us in a given
case ; for example, to regard as an intellectual fact an
idea which is equally a fact of sensibility and a revelation
of will. But it must not be forgotten that this is a service-
able expedient, not a scientifically accurate formulation.

INDEX